The Leather Contest Guide

The Leather Contest Guide

A Handbook for Promoters,
Contestants, Judges
And Titleholders

Guy Baldwin

Daedalus Publishing Company

2nd Edition 2004

Published by
Daedalus Publishing Company
2140 Hyperion Ave.
Los Angeles, CA 90027
USA
http://www.daedaluspublishing.com
323-666-2121

Library of Congress Catalog Card Number: 93-070456

ISBN 1-881943-08-9

Cover photo courtesy of the Leather Archives & Museum

Printed in the United States of America

This book is dedicated to all
those who long for a leather
lifestyle but still live
in secrecy and fear about it.

ACKNOWLEDGEMENTS

Much of this book was written on airplanes during the 29 round trips (38,000 miles) that took me to 24 cities for the 73 different appearances I made as Mr. National Leather Association 1989 and International Mr. Leather 1989 from May, 1989 through October, 1990.

At the 30 contests I participated in during this period, I saw many things done well and done poorly. I met lots of wonderful people as well as a few of the other kind. Among these people were contestants, promotion staff, judges, other titleholders, audience rowdies, bar owners, vendors, and club members; all had something to teach me, and my first thanks must be to all of them.

Special thanks go to Race Bannon who supported me superbly in my bid for both titles and who taught me to write with a computer—a skill without which I never would have learned to write anything. Susie Shepherd, International Ms. Leather 1989, helped with much needed editing and proofing; promotor/sponsors Tony DeBlase and Chuck Renslow provided encouragement, moral support and some very important suggestions, and other material; and producer/director Audrey Joseph who corrected several omissions. My thanks to all these and others who have helped beyond measure.

Race Bannon, Will Russell, Mikal Bales, Chris Hanson, Stephen Darrow, Michael Pereyra, Susie Shepherd, Brian Dawson and others loved me through it all somehow, and I owe them a great deal.

Lastly, I owe immeasurable thanks to my father in leather and first mentor, James Kane, who taught me the value of integrity and honor in all things.

TABLE OF CONTENTS

INTRODUCTION 11

OVERVIEW 13

WHY HAVE A CONTEST? 15

ABOUT THE CONTESTS THEMSELVES 17

PRODUCING THE CONTEST 19

The Early Decisions · Ideas To Consider · Selecting The Date · About Location · Things To Consider About A Bar · Non-Bar Events · Special Considerations with Non-Bar Settings · Negotiations for Non-Bar Settings · Contest Financing · Financing Bigger Events · Finding Contestants And Prizes · Who Makes The Show Happen? · Sample Production Calendar · About The Script · Basic Script Elements · The Usual Script Extras · Fantasy Production · Something New In Fantasies · General Production Tips · Contestant Management · About Emcees · Judges, Judging, and Scoring · How Many Judges? · Special Issues Regarding Judges' Ethics · Personal Arrangements for Judges (or Proper Care and Feeding of Judges) · Scoring The Contestants · Interview vs. Prejudging—A Distinction With A Difference · What Is The Interview? · Scoring for Smaller Contests · The Olympic System

WINNING THE LEATHER CONTEST 71

How To Prepare Yourself For Competition · About Your Body · Being Nearly Nude · Your Stage Skills · What You Have To Say · About Judging · Fantasy Issues And Design · The Winning Edge

JUDGING METHODS AND ISSUES 91

The Judging Sequence · The Interview (May Also Be An Elimination) · The Casual Wear Walk On · Jockstrap/Skinshow · The Fantasy · The "Pop" Question · Full Leather And Speech · Scoring Tips And Ideas · Judging Etiquette

HOLDING A TITLE 103

A Perspective · Some Thoughts On Being A "Leather Star" · Photos And Stationery · Giving Your Autograph · Dealing With Promoters · Wearing Medal And Sash · Tips For Traveling · Small Things That Can Make A Big Difference · About Contests · Issues · A Word About Leadership · A Meditation About Glory

CONCLUSION 121

APPENDIX 123

A Sample Memo to Contestants from Contest Promoter
B Sample Memo to Judges from Contest Promoter
C Sample Judging Form
D Sample Score Elimination Form (Olympic Scoring)
E Sample Judging Procedures and Rules
F Sample Staging Information for Contestants
G Sample Judging Outline
H Sample Contestant Schedule
I Sample Press Release
J Sample Fantasy Script
K Sample Prop List for Fantasy
L Sample Stage Layout for Fantasy

ABOUT THE AUTHOR 141

INTRODUCTION

Currently, the leather contest is the only semi-systematic way we all have with which to identify and encourage local, regional, national, and international leather community leadership. This contest method is perhaps not the ideal way to choose our leadership, but it is "state-of-the-art" for now. Given this, it is important that contests be conducted with style, dignity and intelligence. And, of course, they should be a good time.

Our community deserves the best of the best. If we don't do a good job with our contest system, we are cheating ourselves, and the time for doing that must come to an end. Our community has had second class status in the eyes of many people for far too long; that, too, must change.

This guide has been written to assist contest promoters, contestants, judges and titleholders with respect to the various problems that each of these faces. It has been written with both large and small contests in mind. An effort has been made to use gender-neutral pronouns so that what follows will be useful to all. If you want to hold a contest, you will have many questions about financing, publicity, judging, entertainment, nudity, and a host of other things about which this handbook can advise you.

If you wish to compete, this handbook will help, too. You will find tips about contest preparation: it tells you how good contests are run, explains what the judges tend to be looking for, makes suggestions about how to behave on and off stage, and untangles other questions about the process.

Judges also have special challenges when faced with competent and well-prepared contestants. The section on judging offers judges ideas about how to organize evaluations to help choose the best people for the job.

Lastly, the titleholders themselves have a tough job and are expected to know everything about everything, usually with little or no experience. Lots of great things can be done with a title and the titleholder section is loaded with ideas as well as tips on travel and leather politics.

There is, of course, no guarantee that this book covers everything, but if you pay attention to the issues this book raises, you are much less likely to have the kinds of problems that contests, contestants, judges and titleholders everywhere have suffered from at one time or another.

OVERVIEW

For some time now, leather folks have been gathering for contests where judges select the contestant they feel represents the rest of us in positive ways. Each year, hundreds of contestants compete for the attention of judges and audiences nationwide, and a few winners are chosen for another year.

For various reasons, the idea of organizing, entering, or winning a contest is appealing and exciting, but when we start getting into the nuts and bolts of the thing, we quickly discover that there can be more to it than meets the eye at first glance. Even though there is a lot to organizing a well-run contest, or winning one, that is no reason not to go for it.

The "wing it" method makes for a less-than-wonderful experience and useful opportunities can be lost. If you follow the suggestions made in this book, I can't guarantee you a wild success, but chances are much better that you will be able to avoid problems that have caused others to stumble.

GOOD LUCK!

WHY HAVE A CONTEST?

Contests can be great ways to raise money for a charity, make money for a business, bring business into a bar, bring attention to a club or organization or maybe just offer something new to do.

In addition to all those obvious benefits, contests also offer a chance for various organizations to learn to work together on a project. In places where there has been political infighting, a contest whose purpose is to raise money for a hospice can provide people with an excuse to set their differences aside. Contests can be good opportunities for rivals to have fun together and maybe do some healing.

They also provide an opportunity for vendors and other leather-related businesses to do some advertising. At the same time, the leather community can use contests to show non-leather folks that we are a force to be reckoned with—that we can mobilize both volunteer and financial support for community-related projects that affect us all.

Certainly another bonus of contests is that they create a setting in which leather folks can try their hand at community leadership. Contests are one forum from which leaders emerge. They also give community leaders platforms from which important messages about lifestyle, politics, and sex in the '90s can be gotten out into the community.

These are a few of the ideas that have resulted in successful events in some parts of the country. Maybe they make sense where you are.

ABOUT THE CONTESTS THEMSELVES

These days, for men, there are really two "divisions" or "leagues" of leather contests. One is the International Mr. Leather-type ("IML") contest, and the other is the Mr. Drummer series of contests.

There are some important distinctions between these two types of contests. To enter the Mr. Drummer International contest, usually held in September in San Francisco, one must first enter and win one of the regional Mr. Drummer contests. These contests, including the international finals, must include what is called a "fantasy" segment during the competition—that is, the performance on stage of an erotic leather/SM/fetish skit.

The IML style contest requires no such fantasy segment. Additionally, the winner of the Mr. Drummer International contest is expected to sign a letter of understanding with respect to his obligations and responsibilities; the winner of the IML contest signs no such agreement.

At the International Mr. Leather contest, competitors may be previous winners from cities, states, regions, countries, or they may enter by being sponsored by any lifestyle-related club, organization, or business. These last need never have competed previously to enter the IML competition. This event takes place in Chicago on Memorial Day weekend.

Historically, the Mr. Drummer title has been seen as providing a primarily erotic role model, and the IML title has been viewed as being more about leather community leadership, politics and representation. In recent times, these distinctions have sometimes begun to blur because some Mr. Drummer winners have been interested in representation and politics during the same year that the IML winner had less interest in these responsibilities, and vice versa.

Yet clearly, the Mr. Drummer title has a more well-defined emphasis on the sexuality of the contestant owing to the fact that all contestants (including those competing at the regional level) must perform an erotic fantasy and must agree to appear in an explicit photo spread on the pages of Drummer magazine.

The IML title is the older of the two. Local and regional qualifying contests for both "divisions" generally occur throughout the year prior to the international events themselves.

For women, there is only one "division" so to speak. Although there are many women's leather contests held around the country (none I know of overseas), the contest that is the "grandmother" of them all is the International Ms. Leather ("IMsL") contest. Any woman may enter without having previously won a leather title anywhere else, but all contestants must perform a fantasy as part of the competition. The contest is usually held in the Spring in San Francisco.

Since the issues for contest production, competition, judging and title holding in all three divisions are essentially the same, the following remarks are designed to serve in both divisions.

PRODUCING THE CONTEST

The Early Decisions

Once you have decided to consider launching a contest, there are several main questions to be dealt with right at the beginning. The answers to these will guide your subsequent decision-making.

Probably the first thing to be answered is "What do I/we want to accomplish by holding this contest?" Unless you keep the answer to this question firmly in mind, you are likely to make some painful, and perhaps expensive, social, political and financial turns down the road.

If your purpose is to get more business into your bar on Wednesday nights, then you might want to think about a small event that happens every week to produce a regular week-night crowd. Or you might want to have monthly preliminary contests, the winners of which would compete against each other for the bar's annual leather title. The winner could enter the regional or international event.

On the other hand, you might decide that the local AIDS food bank, or the local gay paper, or some other valuable local organization is in trouble and, "Let's do a contest to bail them out." In these cases, it is easier to enlist the kind of local support that mounting a major offensive on wallets usually requires.

There is, of course, the possibility that you simply want to give the leather folks in the area a chance to come together to meet each other and have a good time while getting to look at some beef for an evening. Fun is always just as valid a purpose as any other!

The bigger the contest, the more people it takes to pull it off. In general, you can get people to donate their time to help with the contest if money is being raised for a charity. If you are trying to make money or promote a business, the members of the support staff who have major responsibilities will usually expect to be paid.

Ideas To Consider

It is better to have a smaller, successful event than a large flop. Events have reputations. A successful event is one that people will remember and want to come back to again and again. It may take three years of smaller events to develop a community to the point where it is ready and able to support a bigger undertaking.

Once an event has been successful, keep the same name and date for the event next time. If the event fails, it is wise to rename, relocate or reposition it on the calendar so that you can get around any bad memories your potential audience may have. This way, you get a second chance with the same audience.

Remember not to bite off more than you can chew. Keep the event in scale with your time, budget, skills, human resources and interest. Otherwise, you will hate the experience and not want to have any part of it again; when this happens, everybody loses. Trying to pull people in at the last moment to save the day does not usually work out well. They will say, "Why didn't you ask me for my help weeks ago when I could easily have scheduled this into my life and been happy to help you out?"

Remember also that the more ambitious the event, the more it is a joint effort—there is more give and take about the decisions, rather than one person dictating how things will go. This is all the more true when the event is a benefit. If you are not a person who works well on a team, the big contest fund raising events might not be for you unless you are willing to pay your help. Big events generally require the skills of team players.

If you are committed to producing a full-blown, well done contest with a smooth and classy presentation that will really make an impression on your community, then I recommend that you go with the "network" system of making it happen. This means assembling a production team and will involve many more people. Strong leaders in the community can accept a chunk of the responsibility more easily than taking on the whole project themselves. Doing things this way has the advantage of spreading the responsibility. It gives more people a chance to become involved who may be looking for a chance at community involvement but don't want to get in over their heads.

This approach also helps the leather community do more outreach in the vicinity and gets the word of mouth out to a much broader base. This can mean increased ticket sales and perhaps even more offers to donate needed help or materials. Since the contest "idea" has become increasingly popular, the leather public is coming to expect more and more from contest productions. Don't be afraid to use this team method to get the job done. If information goes smoothly up and down the chain of command, there will be fewer problems than you might imagine.

Selecting The Date

Location and date are two of the most important early decisions you will make about your event. Do this carefully!

Try to be politically smart when making decisions about the event. Try not to annoy the people whose support you need to make the event a success. For example, it is not a good idea to schedule the event on the same weekend that an important bike club is having its famous annual out-of-town run. The local media won't place your display ads in the best spots if your event conflicts with your town's major annual fund-raising shindig.

Also, with respect to the selection of a date, remember that the national leather publications are anxious to publicize your event for you, but they must be given ample time to do so. Call them and find out when their deadlines are for their calendar sections. This is also a good time to become aware of any conflicts that may exist with other events. Whoever ends up with publicity responsibilities should be warned about publication deadlines, or your event will miss a chance for national attention.

One other factor that may influence the timing of your event might be whether you want your winner to be in a position to compete effectively in the next level of competition, usually IML, Mr. Drummer International, or IMsL. If you have your local contest two weeks before a big international event, your winner's head may still be spinning from the local victory and performance at the next level can sometimes suffer.

If this is a consideration, you may wish to plan the event such that your winner gets some quality experience as a titleholder under his or her belt. This can improve your contestant's chances of winning a larger title in a major way. To be effective as a titleholder, your winner will need to learn how to work an audience, present themselves in public, conduct a fundraiser, think creatively on their feet without warning, and so on. These things take practice.

The value of your winner taking a bigger title is that having a national or international titleholder in your town can have tremendous impact on your area both financially and from a community spirit point of view.

About Location

By tradition, contests are held in leather bars. The advantages are that your audience is already accustomed to going there. Bars already have sound systems and some lighting capability. No special permits are required to sell liquor, and there are rest room facilities. It is easy to target your audience with advertising because you can make announcements about the event for weeks in advance and place posters wherever they will get attention (even over urinals and toilets!).

There are several potential problems to be considered with a bar location. Can the bar hold a big enough crowd to make the event worthwhile? Will there be enough parking? Can you get people to come out for a special event "to the same ol' place"? Can you install a workable stage with the necessary backstage space and dressing rooms? Can you realistically expect patrons to buy a ticket to get into a place they are used to walking into at no charge?

Since many people view bar contests as a gimmick to put more money in the bar owner's pocket, it often happens that other bars will actively not support the contest because it looks like competition for dollars. Several cities I visited as International Mr. Leather were nearly paralyzed by what I have come to call "bar wars"—not exactly what the leather community needs most right now. If the title is not a bar title, it is very wise to host related events at other bars to spread the business around and not make enemies.

Likewise, if the event is held outside of any bar, it is usually possible to get the support of all the local bars, especially if there will be enough time after the contest for the usual weekend bar hopping that goes on.

Quite often, the leather bars available in a particular city are too small to adequately host a major contest. This might be a good time to consider using a non-leather bar or disco just for this one event. This can create a "neutral" space that the various factions of a leather community can more comfortably support, and you can avoid charges of favoritism.

Most discos will at least be willing to discuss the possibility provided their usual heavy business hours won't be affected. This might mean holding the contest earlier than usual so that the crowd can be out before the hour rolls around that the disco really starts humming.

Things To Consider About A Bar

If you do hold the contest in a bar, think about changing the bar in a dramatic way that is low-cost and easy to do, so that patrons feel like something special and different is happening. This can sometimes be done by hanging large pieces of cloth, foil, clear plastic wrap, or other materials from the ceiling. Check fire regulations before such redecorating. If you aren't artsy, get your designer friends to consult. (They'll be flattered with your trust, and you may help them create a special fantasy—who knows?) Special lighting can change a place dramatically, and can be bought or rented. Remember, a contest is largely an entertainment opportunity as far as many people are concerned.

Non-Bar Events

Contests for bar titles, of course, almost always must be held in the bar. In the last few years, there has been a trend toward holding state, regional, national and international contests in non-bar settings like warehouses, theaters, big discos, convention centers and such. In these situations, careful advance planning is required to raise enough money to meet the extra costs that usually go with these larger scale operations to avoid going "in the red." If done carefully, the rewards are great. It is very satisfying to see a big event come off well and benefit a worthy cause.

Non-bar contests can be used to create the impression of a very special event. People are therefore willing to buy a ticket where otherwise they might not. It is usually possible to carry on several other fund-raising activities during the contest in a lobby, or in an adjoining room (silent auctions, art shows or bondage sculpture exhibitions, for example) that are more difficult in bar settings.

Since the staging in non-bar situations is usually so much more comfortable due to added roominess, the producer/director (see definitions below) is often more willing to take bigger risks to offer a more flashy contest and entertainment than would be possible in a bar. Contestants will almost always take these events more seriously and tend to work harder to win. This makes for a more interesting event from the audience point of view.

Non-bar settings offer the chance to hold a "before-the-event" cocktail party on the premises, and (depending on licensing) some other event afterwards—maybe a dance, buffet, bike show, slave auction, carnival, a vendor's alley, a whipping booth, an art show, a bondage sculpture exhibition—or all of the above. This way, patrons get to feel that their ticket bought them several things. The more extras there are, the greater the likelihood that the event will become a big deal that people just won't want to miss ever again, providing it is all well planned and delivered.

Special Considerations with Non-Bar Settings

You might think about providing security guards (maybe you want to call them "monitors"). Many cities have uniform clubs that might happily volunteer for this job if approached about the possibility, or there may be a gay or leather-owned and operated security guard company in your area—check around.

It is a good idea to consult about the event with the local vice squad or police liaison if your city has one, so that the authorities won't be caught off guard by the event. They hate being surprised by these things. It is wise to assume they will find out about it if you don't tell them first. The authorities are more likely to be a problem if they think you have something to hide than if you are up front with them.

This is also the best time to find out exactly what restrictions exist in your city regarding nudity (don't forget to do this!). No place I know of allows any genital nudity. Women usually must have their nipples covered at all times, although some localities allow bare nipples if the audience is maintained at a specified distance from the performer.

As for men, some jurisdictions require a one inch (or more) coverage up the backside, while others permit bare-assed presentations with no rear coverage. Check it out carefully. If law enforcement in your area is itching for an excuse to make trouble, this is an easy one to get nailed on. One photograph is worth a conviction and maybe the loss of liquor licenses. The blow to the morale of a community could be devastating, and recovery a long process. Be sure to inform your contestants about the restrictions so there are no surprises during the contest.

Also, it won't hurt to find out how the authorities feel about uniforms (especially police or highway patrol types) in public. Some jurisdictions have rules about the possession of handcuffs, night sticks, real badges and other police paraphernalia. Leather bar owners will sometimes learn about these things the hard way, so they can be consulted, but a call to the local police captain should answer most of these questions, or consult an attorney.

Many police departments have officers who have volunteered to work gay events in the past. These are good people to hire for your event provided that you explain to them what will happen—the police hate secrets. They tend to be more cooperative when you mention fund-raising efforts first. Hiring off-duty officers to monitor your event is probably the easiest way to avoid confrontations with the authorities or troublesome and unwanted visitors.

Negotiations for Non-Bar Settings

The owner of the building will likely want to know what you are up to. You will get farther by saying that it is a fund raising event to help charity (if true). If there will be fantasies, call them skits—it's a word that will mean the same thing to strangers. You might want to show them a carefully edited version of the videotape from an IML or Mr. Drummer contest.

Nearly all site managers and owners are very reassured if you have hired off-duty police for security. Owners want to know that their place will be left in the same shape as you found it. Send your best diplomats to do this negotiation. Offer a security deposit if that will help. If you plan to book big name entertainment, say so.

Some owners get scared when they see or hear "leather" because they often associate it with punkers, hard rockers or skinheads, any of whom may have caused trouble or damage in the past. Be sure to distinguish yourselves from these groups early during the negotiations.

In general, owners usually have their own standard rental agreements for events. It should have a list of what facilities are included. Find out specifically what equipment is included and excluded in the rental fee. Is it in good working condition? If not, will the rent be reduced? Do you have to hire their people to run it? What is the charge for their staff?

Will there be an owner's representative on hand during the event to solve any equipment problems that may come up and to work with owner's staff? (Most producers have said they think having an owner's representative on hand is a good idea to insist on, especially if there is lots of specialized equipment in the rental deal that could malfunction.) Is there a charge for such a person, or is it included in the rental charge? Develop your questions before you meet with owners and site managers. Don't do this alone; use your key staff and have meetings about it.

Find out about parking, electrical capacity, neighborhood sound restrictions, how early and how late you are allowed to occupy the site, and easy truck access to the space. Some spaces have occupancy limits. Are telephones nearby? How well is the area lit at night—is it safe? Ask the police about the neighborhood at night. Is outside security necessary? If the facility is large, ask what other events might be going on next door—a high school dance, or Rotary Club meeting maybe?

Will your group be responsible for cleanup? If so, to what extent? Is it a simple pick-up of glasses and bottles, or a major vacuuming and rest room scrub down? If you are responsible, build a cleanup staff into your planning. Check with the rental agent to learn if your rental runs into the next day for cleanup, or if your clean-up crew will have to work into the wee hours to satisfy this aspect of the rental contract.

Many of the larger venues may have a surcharge for using video cameras or for selling T-shirts and programs, even if it is a fundraiser. Union places may also require that your ticket sales come through their box office and take a fee. There can also be an extra charge for a live band as opposed to a "track date"—one where all the music comes from a recorded sound track. The general consensus is to avoid dealing with unions because costs and problems have a way of spiraling out of control.

Rental negotiations often include discussion about a percentage of the door, or a percentage of the bar on top of the rental fee. Find out what sorts of rental options the owner will consider, then have a private meeting with your advisors and then get back to the owner with your proposal. This way you don't get rushed into an agreement that you might regret later. Also, the responsibility for making the rental arrangements with the site owners becomes a shared responsibility.

During negotiations, always ask about rehearsal time and whether there are special costs that go with it (like their sound and light technicians). The tendency is to think about the time for the show itself, and forget about set-up, rehearsal and tear-down time. In fact, you will definitely need to have access to the space well before show time; this must be part of the contract. Don't make the mistake of omitting this element from negotiations!

All this negotiating should certainly result in a written contract. Be sure that your negotiators go in with a list of questions, and that notes are made during the conversations. Check the contract to make sure that it reflects your understanding of the particulars. Lock the owners into a date, and find out under which circumstances they may cancel at the last minute—these are usually limited to acts of nature and war and such, but be sure to protect yourself against the owner's last-minute cold feet.

Lastly, think about this. Ideal locations for these kinds of events are not abundant. When you find one that works out really well, don't screw up your relationship with the owners or the space may not be available again next year. If the location owner/manager sees that you run a tight ship and have your staff organized and know what you need and how to handle yourself, you are much more likely to get cooperation when it comes time to start planning next year's event which, hopefully, you will do early.

Contest Financing

In general, the smaller the contest, the easier it is to finance. Weekly or monthly bar contests are usually held during the week and rely on facilities that are already in place. At minimum, it doesn't take more than a good microphone and a skilled emcee to do a fairly straightforward contest that can be a good time and generate income. In these cases, there is almost no extra cost involved unless you decide to run some display ads in local gay papers and/or businesses, or mail out a batch of flyers.

Since most bar contests have the purpose of generating business for the bar owners, any costs are considered business expenses related to advertising, so usually financing these is no problem.

Most often, you can find local people to act as judges, so you don't have the costs associated with bringing in celebrity titleholders from other cities. On the other hand, if you want to draw a big crowd, you might want to consider booking one or more well-known titleholders or other leather celebrities (publishers, photographers, artists, columnists, vendors, etc.) to come in for your event. It is a very good idea to use his/her name and photos on the advance publicity to generate interest.

Here and there, a bar owner wants to make a name for the bar in the leather community and stages a more serious contest to find a real contender for a major title. If the bar's titleholder wins the bigger event, the titleholder can be used for promotional purposes and potentially make the bar's name a household word during travels as a major titleholder. This tends to be good for business, but such a contest itself can be more expensive to mount.

Unless there are major titleholders in the area who can be available to serve as judges, one might be brought in (finances allowing) to bring some prestige to the event and the title. These days, this is not usually a problem because there are now reputable titleholders nearly everywhere. Don't hesitate to use last year's or the year before's winner. Also, there are many very well-known leather celebrities who are not titleholders and who are very experienced judges.

It takes a sizable crowd and good contest management to create respect for a title. The advertising to bring in a big crowd might cost a bit more. The more you do to make your event a big deal, the more it costs, but the more the promoter stands to gain if it comes off well.

Remember, a small success is better than a big flop!

Financing Bigger Events

Unless you happen to be Mr. Gotbucks, doing a bigger event is going to cost more than the average bar show. All or most of the services normally found in a bar, sometimes including a liquor license, must be rented or borrowed. Costs go up when you create something from nothing.

This sort of event is usually financed by a group of people who have an interest in seeing it happen. Generally, somebody decides to circulate a letter asking who is interested in a preliminary meeting, and then one is scheduled. This might include a group of leather-related business owners or clubs (bars, leather shops, bike clubs, lifestyle organizations).

Typically, they know that their city is ready to support a big event, but individually, they know they don't have the money or hands to make it happen. Usually, businesses have money but no hands, and organizations have hands but little money, so in theory, they can only make it happen together.

In preliminary discussions, it is very important for everybody to say what they want for themselves or their organizations out of the event, and to say what they can offer to the success of the event. Only when all these cards are on the table does everybody get to find out what resources are available and which ones need to be chased down.

Nobody does something for nothing. Even satisfaction is a worthy payoff to many people for effort expended. Things tend to work much more smoothly when everybody can be honest and up-front about what exchanges they are willing to participate in.

These preliminary meetings should make it possible to develop two resource lists: one for how much money is available, and the second for how much people power is available. These facts will determine the size and scale of the event that will be possible by using the available dollar and human resources.

This process can be fairly simple and straightforward if people are willing to approach these discussions with an open mind and understand that there is more than one right way to do these kinds of events. The danger arises when people stop being flexible and fail to keep their "eye on the prize," so to speak.

Ideally, these meetings will have taken place at least six months before the event is likely to occur. Before any commitments are made for booking anything or anybody, there should be clear understandings about who is going to pay for what and when that payment is expected to happen. It must also be made clear what the "people power" commitments will be as planning goes forward. These events work best when they are run as businesses.

If it looks like money may be short, perhaps some preliminary fundraising can fix the problem. Sunday brunches or afternoon beer busts, raffles, leather swap meets, open workshops/demos on leather-related topics and such can all be offered to the leather public for a donation to help raise money for organizations that need extra dollars to launch the event.

It may be possible to raise money by selling advance advertising to local businesses which could appear in a program to be printed. If you go this route, plan ahead carefully so that deadlines for copy can be met easily. Be sure to include some "editorial copy" from the producers, celebrity titleholders and the beneficiary charity in the program so it doesn't just look like a packet of advertising. Don't forget to contact businesses that are not located in your area but who do a big mail order trade. They will often take out ads even though they have no local store.

One financial strategy that has paid off handsomely in several places is to give businesses the chance to underwrite specific parts of the event. One way to do this is to make a list of the elements that you think the event really needs to make it happen. Then assign an estimated dollar value to each of these. Once you have such a list, it is much easier to go to a specific potential donor and say, "How would you like to help us out by subsidizing the flowers at the such-and-such part of the event; we think it will cost $1,500.00, and that would help us out a great deal?"

If that is more money than the donor can afford, then you can offer him/her the chance to do something else that you think will cost less. When discussing this, indicate that you will list the donors in the program. In this way, you can get specific funds for a headline entertainer, bringing in a special judge, emcee or disc jockey. You can then announce that this person is, "Here through the generosity of the Black and Blue Bar" or whomever the donor might be.

Remember that organizations can donate warm bodies to help out with various tasks like running the ticket booth at the door, or staffing a no-host bar or filling other such volunteer needs. Again, remember to acknowledge every contribution that comes from individuals, businesses or organizations with at least a letter thanking them for their donation when they commit to it, and another one after the event.

When planning your budget, don't forget to take into account things that can be donated to save (or make) money. For Fantasy '89, Omaha's first-ever leather event which was very successful, T-shirts were donated, the silkscreening on them was donated, enough food for a cook-out buffet was donated, and so was most of the other printing and paper for the event.

Your approach to potential donators will be successful more often if you mention the "benefit" part first. The worst that can happen when you ask for someone to donate something is that people can say, "no"—you're no worse off than you were before you asked.

If your early meetings reveal that no one seems to have emcee skills, then you can think about importing one for the event. Some very successful events have been done with co-emcees so that two, perhaps three people with even some skill at this can combine their efforts to complement each other at the microphone. Since a new era of cooperation between men's and women's leather communities is upon us, there is a trend to have co-emcees—one of each gender and often, former titleholders. There is always a way. The trick is to find that way by using what is available.

Occasionally, it will be possible to line up one major sponsor who will be willing to pay for any expenses that the organizers just can not seem to cover any other way, usually up to a previously agreed upon maximum amount. This sponsor will almost always expect that the name of their business figures prominently in the advertising of the event and is the first to be thanked from the stage.

Finding Contestants And Prizes

To get people to compete in a smaller, local or bar contest, there needs to be an inducement. Raw ego and exhibitionism are often enough in a "just for fun" event, but they don't cut it in a serious contest. That means prizes that count. The prize scale rises commensurately with the scope of the contest.

A weekly "wet shorts contest" (Los Angeles) earns the winner $50.00, and second place $25.00. The bar where this started now has a big crowd regularly on Thursday nights whereas before, they had been rather slow nights. You can talk to local leather makers and maybe get them to donate goods from their shops as prizes in exchange for having their names mentioned from the stage. Remember to mention them, or they won't want to donate their goods again.

The local promoters of events that produce contenders for the big national and international events almost always guarantee air fare and hotel expenses for the local winner who is going on to compete again in the bigger event. That can amount to five or six hundred dollars. In your advance publicity to solicit contestants, be sure to mention the major prizes and what other contest(s) the winner will go on to enter.

Local contest promoters can get contest funding and prize money in several ways: direct payment by the sponsoring organizations or businesses, or by asking local supporters to donate a portion of the prize. Raffles, beer busts, auctions and such are also possibilities.

There is usually a gay or leather-friendly travel agent in most places; cultivate this person. Where there are more than one, spread your opportunities equally between them.

Gay and leather-supportive businesses like unusual opportunities to get their name around because it may mean new markets for them. Restaurants can donate dinner for two, travel agents can donate airfare to a town to which they already may have free tickets, and so on.

A serious bid for a big national or international title is truly a big effort and always costs the contestants money from their own pocket. Usually their inducement to compete is a combination of desire for attention, the prizes, glory, and a real wish to be of service to the community—all in various combinations, depending on the contestant.

Once you know what your prizes will be, you can begin a publicity campaign to solicit contestants. If it's a cash prize for a weekly contest in a bar, that might mean simply having the manager walk around to the bar patrons who have gathered and talk people into entering by mentioning the $50.00 first prize.

If it is the bar's annual contest, you might want to circulate flyers a month or two before the show. This could include sending flyers to the local bike clubs, leather shops and kinky organizations to see if they want to enter one or more of their members. Such flyers should always mention the prizes.

In smaller towns, be sure to include some comments about what will be involved in entering as a contestant, because people are sometimes too embarrassed to admit they don't know how to enter a contest, even though they might want to. Help your potential contestants out with this information.

The ad placed in the local gay paper can mention who contestants should contact if they want to enter or just want more information. Local leather-related businesses should all be contacted for prize solicitation and to be given the chance to offer their own candidate.

Who Makes The Show Happen?

Making a contest come off smoothly is a task that can rest on the shoulders of just one person, as often happens in smaller contests, or it can be shared by a committee of any size, with one person bearing ultimate responsibility. As in all things, the less you try to pull off, the easier it will be to make the show happen. Or, the more you try, the harder you will have to work, and maybe you can't do it all by yourself.

When we start to consider the larger (state, regional, national and international) contests, then it is necessary for many people to be involved to get the jobs done. Just what are the jobs? Who does what?

In a way, a contest is simply a specialized form of staged entertainment with the added feature that a leather contest happens in and around the entertainment. In the smaller contests, the contestants themselves are the entertainment. If leather contests were not entertaining, people would have less interest in them.

In a sense, the contest is really between the contestants and the judges. Technically, the audience isn't really even necessary for a winner to be chosen. You don't have to like this, but it is important to understand. Having an audience there is fun for the contestants, and can help raise money. But unless there is something in it for the audience, folks will get bored and start complaining and then leave, perhaps never to go to another contest.

Because a contest is built around entertainment, most jobs are the same as on any entertainment stage. Here are some jobs that go with the big contests. Smaller contests are less complex, but they have similar roles and similar goals and problems.

Executive Producer—In a privately-owned contest like Mr. Drummer or IML, this person usually provides the cash and some ideas about what s/he wants to see happen in the show. The Executive Producer may be involved in the major artistic decisions, but generally leaves the "nuts and bolts" operations to assistants. In group efforts, this is often the chair of the contest committee, whose basic job is as an overseer and coordinator.

Producer/Director or Co-Producers—This person (or persons) actually wears several hats. S/he has administrative, financial and artistic responsibility for the show. S/he selects the principal assistants who, all together, will create the result that will pack the place and satisfy those who come to watch.

The Producer/Director must direct the ideas and activities of lighting, sound, stage crew people, contestants, speakers, and entertainment to produce a satisfying event, and also work out the script with the Executive Producer.

This person meets personally with the on-site manager of the facility where the show is held once the place has been rented. It is he or she who usually makes arrangements to rent the location.

After that, s/he works closely with the staff of the location.

The Producer/Director also attends to many of the non-artistic details of the show either directly or through assistants. These things might include: negotiating group rates with hotels and airlines for out-of-towners; arranging ground transportation for celebrities, judges and other VIPs; making sure that lunch is provided during rehearsals; designing judging forms; working with concessions; overseeing ticket sales; registering contestants; deciding seating arrangements, if any; possibly even driving a bus.

This is the person who also must ensure that the contestants are where they are supposed to be on time, every time, and may also arrange for pickup and delivery of any special props that may be required for the show.

The Producer/Director (or Co-Producer) has a big job. At the big, private events, s/he functions as the Producer, Director and Technical Director and often calls all the cues during the event itself and does the hiring of equipment and operators.

When the show is a group effort, the jobs of Producer, Director, and Technical Director are sometimes held by different people who are all members of the contest committee and report to the chair.

Publicity—This person is responsible for advertising the event. S/he designs posters, flyers, display ads and press releases for local newspapers, and writes any radio or TV advertising. S/he may write articles that hype the contest or make announcements in bars. This person may also be in charge of ticket sales. S/he helps plan the date so that no major community conflicts happen. In short, if no one comes, this one is in deep water. This job is sometimes done by several people with a chairperson to oversee a "to do" list. Remember to check the publication deadlines of national media so your event will be listed. Many of those wanting to attend will need lots of advance notice to budget time and money for it.

If there is to be a souvenir program, Publicity might sell ads to vendors who want display advertising. This raises some money to defray the cost of mounting the show. Sometimes a Co-Producer does these jobs.

Business and Finance—This person is responsible for developing budgets and restraining others from overspending. S/he may be in charge of bank accounts and ticket sales and is expected to prepare a balance sheet after the event.

If there is a fundraising component to the event, it is crucial that very careful records of income and expenditures be kept, because elements in the community may raise hell if they suspect money was mishandled. In fact, it may be well to consider that more than one senior member of the production team be involved in decisions to spend more than a specified amount, so that the event managers don't find themselves the subject of a local scandal.

In some communities, the politics are so complex that somebody may be waiting for a chance to stir up trouble. Careful record-keeping and cash control is your best defense against these problems. Consider publishing an abbreviated balance sheet in the local paper after the event.

Stage Manager—Has authority backstage and manages the stage crew backstage. Supervises movement of large props, scenery, scrims, curtains, risers, podiums, etc. and is usually responsible to the Director or Producer/Director, as the case may be.

Contestant Manager—This is the production team's representative to the contestants. This job is so important that an entire section is devoted to its explanation below.

Judge Coordinator—This is the production team's representative to the judges. This job is also an important one that is described in detail below.

Sample Production Calendar

Below is a sample "To Do" list for a major contest with most of the frills and extras. Some things can be done earlier, and a few can be done later than recommended. The list is not complete, and you will think of other items. This will just get you thinking in terms of a rough calendar. Doing things at the last minute makes people crazy. Plan ahead and save yourself unnecessary stress.

If what you want to do is not so grand as all this, just eliminate the things on the list that don't apply to your situation. If you plan to do other types of things (auctions, carnivals, etc.) during the contest, those things also need to be worked into your master calendar. Such a calendar is most useful when it is constantly updated and there is good follow-up to confirm that things really are completed as promised and on schedule.

To Do List For Contest Production

(*To be completed as early as possible; preferably, 6-8 months before event*)

- Make decisions about size, scale, and purpose of contest.
- Begin master list of names, addresses, telephone numbers of all who will be involved in event production, in alphabetical order.
- Check on local nudity regulations.
- Check on local liquor regulations.
- Check on local fire and special effects regulations (fire, smoke or flashpots on stage).
- Contact local law enforcement agencies.
- Are special permits needed?
- Special event insurance needed? Available? Rules?
- Evaluate available locations with above answers in mind.
- Select Producer and assistants (provide with phone list).
- Select Director and assistants (provide with phone list).
- Form a production committee (key personnel). Make a meeting schedule for this group and provide members with name and phone list.

- Key personnel should visit potential sites to evaluate them.

- Decide on the Location.

- Choose Date. Coordinate with other events and site availability and schedules of key personnel. Check titleholder availability for judging and emceeing and the schedule of the charity to benefit from the contest proceeds, if any.

- Notify other community leaders of your intention and date.

- Book the selected location.

- Negotiate group rates & bookings with hotels and airlines.

- Contact and book possible judges and titleholders.

- Book, or at least begin the search for, entertainers.

(*To be completed at least 3 months before event*)

- Collect phone lists from key personnel, merge and update, then print and redistribute them.

- Solicit bids for program publication & select printer.

- Coordinate any vendors who may be involved.

- Establish deadlines for advertisers and titleholders to submit ad copy and editorial copy for program.

- Contact potential prize donors. Get prize commitments.

- Make logo and other "image" decisions for public relations use.

- Prepare publicity campaign. Consult with the production committee.

- Notify media with press releases. Get their advertising deadlines.

- Arrange for ticket printing.

- Contact local security firm for rates and other related info.

- Prepare mailing lists for announcement of the event to relevant clubs. Generate announcements, and mail.

- Establish advanced ticket mail-out deadline.

- Prepare materials to accompany mailed tickets or ticket confirmations which includes event information: hotels, restaurants, vendors, related or other events happening in town, and preliminary schedule for the weekend or event.

(*To be completed at least 2 months before event*)

- Update & copy phone lists; redistribute to key personnel.

- Commission commemorative pins, buttons, mugs, T-shirts, winners' trophies, winners' medals and such.

- Write contestant application forms & distribute to bars, leather shops, clubs and organizations, and other outlets. Indicate what the categories of competition will be and give some information about how the contest will be scored.

- Begin contestant outreach to encourage entrants.

- Remind advertisers and providers of editorial copy about copy deadline for program printing.

- Arrange for photographer for event.

- Arrange any special production equipment or props.

(*To be completed at least 1 month before event*)

- Collect, update, print, and redistribute phone list to key personnel
- Confirm VIPs and titleholders. Discuss arrival schedules.
- Write script—Director with Producer.
- Arrange transportation needs for contestants and judges—buses, vans, drivers and schedules.
- Inform contestants about guidelines for fantasy production and request fantasy script and music.

(*To be completed at least 3 weeks before the event*)

- Supervise printing of the souvenir program

(*To be completed at least 2 weeks before the event*)

- Schedule rehearsal time.
- Mail final schedule indicating rehearsal schedules and locations to VIP participants and registered contestants. VIPs should be informed about all their required appearances so they can plan accordingly. Inform these people as to which events they are getting complimentary admissions, and which things they will be expected to pay for themselves. List optional events that they may attend if they wish. Please make clear indications about whether their complimentary admissions include significant others or not.

(*To be completed at least 1 week before the event*)

- Schedule a meeting to take place after the event to include a discussion among all key personnel about how the contest went. Do this now to deflect possible paranoia later if the event should have some serious problem—your staff won't think you're after somebody's hide.

- Make preparations for some sort of "after party" (Afterglow party, Coming down party, Catch your breath ball, whatever) for contestants, judges, key personnel at banquet room or other facility.

- Determine staging (who moves where, when and how on stage).

- Create set-up and tear-down crew schedules for contest day.

- Make decisions about scoring and point counting (the tally process).

- Prepare judging forms.

- Prepare badges for officials, judges, contestants and contestant numbers.

- Prepare advance ticket pickup packets.

- Collect prizes for distribution to winners.

- Prepare information handout for contestants.

- Schedule VIP pickup at airport.

- Arrange for food and beverages to be available during rehearsals and in dressing rooms for contestants, staff, judges and VIPs during the show, as desired.

- Hold a meeting for all key personnel to review areas of responsibility and go over who will do what and when, and who needs to coordinate with whom.

(*To be completed a day or two before the event*)

- Distribute registration packets to advance ticket holders.

- Register contestants and provide them with rehearsal schedule.

- Confirm set-up and tear-down crew schedules.

(*To be completed within two weeks after the event*)

- Meet with all key personnel to review how things went and make suggestions for next year. Initial financial reckoning should be complete for report to committee. This meeting should be tape recorded.

- Thank you letters to: vendors, contestants, judges, key personnel, owners, security firm, prize donors, advertisers, off-duty police.

- Letters of congratulations to the three winners.

- Schedule meeting with winner and key personnel to discuss sponsorship for IML, IMsL, Mr. Drummer or Mr./Ms. National Leather Association ("NLA") finals. (The Mr./Ms. NLA contest is another important national contest.) This is also the right time to explain to the winner what the sponsor expects in terms of participation and such. Sponsors should think about establishing an event calendar and block in the winner's time before s/he gets swamped with other requests.

- Send out press releases and photography of the contest that contain a brief description of the event, perhaps mentioning which VIPs were there, community response, who the winners are and perhaps something about the sponsors, and what charity (if any) benefited and perhaps the amount raised if it was a benefit. Both local and national media should get the press release and copies of photos.

- Rest, Rest, Rest.

About The Script

A script for a contest is basically the recipe for what will happen from the moment the signal is given for the show to start until the audience applause stops after the show is over. Usually, the script is created by the Producer/Director in collaboration with the Executive Producer and whichever assistants they choose to include in the process.

The purpose of the script is to eliminate confusion from the minds of the following people about what is supposed to happen next: Director, Producer, Stage Manager, Lighting and Sound personnel, and Emcee(s) and Contestants. These are the people who control what goes on during the show. They are responsible for organizing people, things, effects, music and lights, so that all action on stage moves smoothly from one part to the next in the proper order and without problems.

In short, the script is the formula for the event. At a small, weekly show, the script may be so simple that it is not even written down. At a bar contest that happens once a month, it may take up no more than a sheet of paper. At a regional, national or international event, it may run to 50 pages of detailed instructions, including light cues and specific directions to stage hands.

When planning scripts for big events, Producers and Directors are wise to keep several things in mind:

- The more complex the script, the more time may be demanded in rehearsal to make it come off smoothly. Have you booked the location for enough days to ensure adequate stage set-up and rehearsal time? Do you need to schedule rehearsals elsewhere a few days earlier for dancers, etc.?

- Very few audiences will tolerate a show lasting more than three hours unless it is truly spectacular. Recently, informal polling at the big international shows has revealed serious audience annoyance with their length. If you must have a long show, consider having it over two days and making the event a big weekend. For the most part, audiences have a very short attention span for almost anything, including dancers, singers and comedians. Generally, there must be some change in the action on stage at least every 90 seconds or so. Important speeches are the usual exception and even they should be limited to ensure audience attention. Four minutes for a speech is a good maximum to shoot for unless your speaker is spellbinding, and even then, the audience won't sit still much longer than four minutes.

- Master scripts should contain light cues, sound cues and movement cues for emcees, and stage cues for stage manager and staff. All participants should be well rehearsed before the final dress rehearsals for continuity, and to discover and fix glitches.

  Master scripts should also contain the remarks the emcees will make about the contestants, i.e. "Jane Jones, from Denver, Colorado is 5'5" tall and weighs 100 pounds, loves wrestling, and is Ms. Colorado Leather, 1990...."

  The Producer/Director usually calls all the cues during the show itself.

- If your script is large (you decide) and your rehearsals and technical rehearsal reveal that you need to make some changes, it can be very handy to have the script on a word processor so that any changes can be made easily, and the new script printed either the night before or day of the show. Doing this saves the Producer/Director from having to make sense out of scribbles in margins during the show under tension and pressure. This also enables each of the principal production people to have a fresh script that is guaranteed to have all the changes in it. Thus, the probability of glitches in the show is minimized.

- These days, contestants are generally required to fill out an application which contains relevant information (astrological birth signs are not necessary). When each contestant is on stage during the first walk-on, and again during the jockstrap/skinshow presentation, various information about the contestant is read to the audience from the application by the emcee(s).

In a large show, it is wise to incorporate these remarks directly into the script to eliminate paper shuffling at the podium by the emcee(s). On occasion, nervous emcees have been known to drop the actual applications and get them out of order which is very confusing to the judges, and it can seriously unnerve the contestants. It breaks their concentration and that of the judges and audience. When a problem like this happens, judges don't see contestants at their best.

Below are the basic, bare bones elements in the leather contest as it has evolved. In some places, there are more elements and in others, fewer. Sometimes the order of these events is changed slightly, and intermissions are not shown—there may not be any, and there may be up to three.

Basic Script Elements

The emcee (usually in this order): (1) welcomes audience; (2) introduces the contestants in street wear (first judging?), explains contest to audience, includes scoring procedures and the importance of the Interview segment; (3) introduces judges (least "senior" first); (4) introduces senior titleholder on judging panel for a speech; (5) introduces contestants again in skimpy wear (second judging); (6) announces individual contestant fantasies to be performed, if any (judged for score); (7) introduces contestants in full leather for speech or questions (last judging); (8) introduces entertainment, if any, while scores are totaled, calls for outgoing titleholder's remarks; (9) calls back all contestants; (10) makes essential thank yous; (11) announces second runner up; (12) announces first runner up; (13) announces winner and the show ends, usually with photo opportunities for winners and others on stage.

Many shows add entertainments, intermissions and announcements to the above formula to fill out the evening and buy time for the contestants to change clothes and get ready for the next segment, or for the judge's scores to be tallied and results determined. Sometimes the amount of extras included can be determined by how many contestants are in the show. In theory, the more contestants, the fewer extras are necessary to add up to a full-sized show.

The chief reason that the big national and international shows have gotten into time problems is that they have more and more contestants and feel obligated to also add many or all of the extras.

The Usual Script Extras

Any of the following can be added to a script: an exciting musical warm-up, often with dancers or a singer; comments about the prizes that have been donated; an opening fantasy performed (titleholder or leather performer); speeches by celebrities sprinkled throughout the script; remarks about the evening's beneficiary charity; remarks about other activities happening on premises or in town; presentation of colors of club representatives present; drawing raffle numbers; a band, comedian, skit or fantasy performance; a dazzling special effect; banter between co-emcees; endless thank yous for all those who made the show happen; a leather fashion show with (or not) the items being auctioned; fifteen leather elephants doing tricks, and others.

The point of the extras is to add interest for the audience while the contestants are readying themselves for whatever is next. The trick with adding extras is to not delay the progress of the contest.

Contestants usually spend a lot of time waiting to go on stage while emcees buy them even more unnecessary and unwanted time.

Fantasy Production

When there are fantasies to be performed, preparing the stage can take some time, but this is usually easily covered by some emcee patter, or by having one fantasy going on in one place while the next one is being set up somewhere else to save time. The Mr. Drummer 1990 contest arranged the script such that a contestant was giving his speech while the stage crew was setting up for the next fantasy—this worked very smoothly.

In some places, producers have also tried to solve this problem by using a split stage—half the stage is being set up for the next fantasy while the other half is used for a fantasy in performance. This can be distracting for the audience and judges unless there is enough visual distance separating the set-up crew from the contestant performing.

Something New In Fantasies

In some situations, there is not enough room to allow for the performance of full scale fantasies. One novel solution to this problem has been used successfully in a contest in Dallas, and that is to have the contestants videotape their fantasy beforehand and have it shown to the audience during the contest.

This allows for the contestant to "go on location," so to speak, and employ material or individuals who might otherwise not be available, even if the stage space were not a problem. The creative possibilities are almost endless, and this also eliminates all the complex stage work that goes with fantasy production. The contestant can stand on stage before, during or after the fantasy and make some remarks about it if so desired by the promoters.

Promoters can rent the necessary equipment to show the video in the bar or wherever for a nominal fee, or someone might be persuaded to bring in their big screen TV for this purpose. Also, the event could be held in a bar where video monitors are already in place.

This fantasy technique makes judging extra tough for several reasons: first, most judges have no experience evaluating video fantasies; second, this method does not allow judges to evaluate how a contestant performs before a live audience; and third, judges may make their point assignments on the basis of a contestant's (or the video's production crew) video production skills rather than the erotic content of the presentation.

This method of bringing fantasies into a contest does require plenty of advance outreach to contestants so that they will have enough time to make the necessary preparations to do the videotaping. If this method were to be used in a prerequisite contest for a larger, national contest, inquiries about its permissibility should first be made to the promoters of that contest.

General Production Tips

Do your very best to have the event begin on time. Those who come late because they expect you to be late will know better next time. Always think about next time. Double-check to make sure that everything works: lights, sound, microphones, etc. The power of an event to draw and satisfy a crowd is lost if the staged presentation looks slipshod. Patrons will then learn that this is nothing special and perhaps not come again in future years.

If at all possible, arrange some kind of rehearsal, especially for the emcee, contestants, and backstage helpers, if any. Give each contestant the chance to use a microphone—many have never had one in their hands, especially at the local contest level. This can be fun to do in a group (the contestants, that is) so they can give each other feedback. Try to have someone really knowledgeable available to help them so that they know how to hold the mike to their best advantage.

At the bigger, more elaborate events, a technical rehearsal has become an absolute must. The more complex a show becomes, the greater the chance for something to go wrong.

Make provisions for key personnel to be able to communicate with each other during the show. I strongly suggest headsets to ease communication problems. These can be rented, and they can make a big difference in how smoothly the show runs. The wireless kind work great outdoors, but might not work indoors due to interference with the sound system. Check this out carefully!
These should be used by the Director, Producer, Stage Manager, Asst. Stage Manager, sound person, light person, and spotlight operators.

During the event, the Producer/Director always has priority air rights, and s/he reads ahead in the script and cues the light, sound, and stage people so that the show goes smoothly.

As your audience arrives, it is a good idea to provide a titleholder sign-up sheet in a conspicuous place so that the emcees can mention their presence. This is a nice courtesy to extend because many titleholders work hard and announcing their support of the present event is a nice way to acknowledge their efforts. Custom in these matters dictates that they be announced in the following order: local titles first, then state, regional, national, then finally, international.

When introducing the judging panel to the audience, it is becoming customary to introduce non-titleholders first, then junior titleholders and finally, the senior titleholders with the most senior titleholder judge being introduced last. S/he usually makes a short speech after his/her introduction.

If the judging and scoring has been carefully planned, it should never take more than 30 minutes to produce the result. (See the section on Judging for detailed suggestions.) If you try to stick to the three-hour time limit suggested above, that means that all your judging is done in two and one-half hours and the tabulation takes up the rest of the time. Plan carefully.

Once the first place winner has been announced, the show is over. It is not a good idea to speak to the audience again from the stage—it spoils their jubilation. The winner should not make any kind of speech now, because his/her thoughts are likely to be a jumble and it is unlikely that a good impression will be made. The emcee should wait until the cheering has gone on for a minute or so, and then dismiss those who did not place to the dressing rooms.

Then, the emcee can step forward to arrange the winners for photo opportunities. The first one should be of all three winners. The next one should be of the first place winner by him or herself. After that, there are many other possibilities which can include: last year's winner congratulating the new winner; the winner with the senior titleholder present; the winner with the judging panel; or the winner with the producer or club officers, as the case may be.

Someone should always accept responsibility for arranging photo opportunities because such a chance will otherwise be lost forever. Do not rely on the winners to do this for themselves because they are in a daze at this point and will need some direction to provide good photographs for the press.

Someone on the production team should be among those taking photos so that they can appear in both local and national press.

Contestant Management

Contestants are very special people and must be treated as such. After all, without contestants, there is no contest. In a certain sense, contestants come from a kind of undefined and unrecognizable pool of contestants who are out there and usually unaware of one another. One can never tell just who might turn up to enter a contest.

For this reason and others, it is very important to treat all contestants well once they identify themselves to you by entering or even talking about the possibility of entering your contest. Those who want to try their hand at contests may know they want to enter, but wait until next year to actually do so. These days, it takes most potential contestants about three to nine months or longer to prepare themselves for the effort—and it is an effort.

If word gets out that you don't treat contestants well, potential contestants will get turned off and perhaps wait to enter a contest until they discover that conditions have improved or until they move to a different city, if they don't lose interest first.

Promoters often can be heard to complain that they can't get people to enter their contest, but these same promoters rarely stop to think that their handling of prior contestants may be the very reason. Promoters must always think about the impact this year's contest will have on the situation in the community and the contestant pool next year, and in the years to come.

In all the really well-run contests, the promoters have a commitment to all contestants to make the experience a good one; win, place or lose. It is wise to keep in mind the fact that a contestant who doesn't win this year, but really wants to serve the community through titleholding, may try again next season. But that contestant will only consider trying again if s/he had a good experience with the competition itself. Just what goes into making the contest a good experience for the contestants?

Most people don't know this, but leather contests (and, I suspect other competitions as well) are very trying experiences in one's life. During the contest, the contestant can often experience a subtle transformation of consciousness, feelings and perspectives. Contestants are grouped together in unusually close, yet highly competitive circumstances, and are expected to do and say things that are very personal in front of large groups of strangers. None of this is easy. Consequently, contestants need specialized assistance to get through the experience.

Often by the end of the contest evening, contestants have been on an emotional roller coaster ride that is unequalled. The subtle transformation accumulates as the event progresses, such that the contestant may feel as though he or she is in a kind of trance by the end of the evening. Most promoters are completely unaware that this process takes place. Most contestants are confused by the experience and may never find words to describe it, even to themselves, and, least of all, to each another.

Following are some recommendations that can ease this process for contestants. These comments are designed for the bigger events and you, the promoter, will have to decide to what lengths you are willing to go to make competition a good experience for competitors, based on how much help you have and how much money you want to spend. Fortunately, doing this particular job right doesn't cost an arm and a leg. Mostly, it just takes some thoughtfulness and a selection of the right person for the job.

The production/organization group needs to include a Contestant Manager, as mentioned above. In most places, this person has come to be known as "The Mother" or "Den Daddy" probably because his/her role is basically one of nurturing, protection, and instruction. S/he may have one or more assistants who will be needed during the event or weekend itself. In the very big shows, there are between three and eight people assigned to these tasks.

The Contestant Manager, along with assistants, is responsible for contestant needs off stage, and the emcees, Stage Manager and/or Producer/Director is responsible for contestant needs on stage.

This person's job is, roughly as follows:

- Prepare a fairly detailed handout for all contestants and see to it that contestants get this handout as soon as their entry is confirmed. The handout (see example in Appendix) should include information about the event that tells exactly where the contestants are supposed to be and when they are supposed to be there. It outlines the sequence of appearances the contestants will be expected to make both before and during the contest, including Prejudging and all rehearsals. It must tell them, in general terms, what they will be expected to wear, and must include any restrictions dictated by the local nudity regulations, as well as restrictions about uniforms, handcuffs, nightsticks, badges, and the like.

Nothing is harder on a contestant than not knowing what is expected of her/him and when it is expected. Learning these things at the last minute can be confusing and disorienting for contestants to the degree that contestants have been known to drop out of a contest at the last minute or even during the competition. Word gets around, and promoters suffer in the contestant department when these complaints filter through the community.

The contestant handout should explain the sequence of the contest and contain information about the points per category to be earned, and perhaps include some comments about Olympic scoring, if it is to be used.

- The Contestant Manager should be introduced to each contestant and told that this is the person who has been assigned to help the contestants with any questions or specialized needs. In contests where fantasies are performed by contestants as part of the competition, the Contestant Manager may have to interface with the Stage Manager and/or the Producer/Director.

- It is usually the Contestant Manager's responsibility to keep the contestants together once they arrive at the place where the contest will take place. The Contestant Manager keeps outsiders out and insiders in with respect to the dressing rooms. They do not typically help the contestants with dressing—by custom, contestants are urged to help each other with this task.

- The Contestant Manager must serve as the advocate for the

contestants with respect to the production team. The Contestant Manager needs to provide private dressing rooms as needed that are equipped with at least one large mirror. Washroom facilities should be close at hand and, preferably, for the exclusive use of the contestants.

- Food and drink during rehearsals and during the contest should be provided for the contestants at no charge, and the Contestant Manager should see to these needs.

- The Contestant Manager ushers the contestants to the wings from which contestants will make their stage entrances. It is wise for the Contestant Manager to have a headset or at least be cued in enough time to get contestants ready to proceed with the contest.

  It is generally a good idea for the Contestant Manager to have a copy of the script to follow and to be able to answer questions the contestants are sure to ask. The Contestant Manager will often give 15, 10, and 5-minute warnings to the contestants and tell them in advance that s/he will be doing so. This helps contestants pace themselves and contain their anxiety about their performance.

- The Contestant Manager should provide numbers to the contestants to be worn when on stage, and contestant badges to be worn when making social (not for official scoring) appearances where judges may be present.

- The Contestant Manager escorts the contestants to and from the room where the interview portion of the judging is to be held, and has the contestants together and ready in time so the judges are not kept waiting.

In short, this job is part therapist, part go-fer, part parent, and part friend. S/he is the production team's personal representative and ambassador to the contestants. Executive Producers should choose people for this job who are fair, cooperative, willing to stick up for the contestants with respect to production team decisions, and have a strong maternal or paternal streak. This is not the place for large egos. The contestants do not need to compete with this person. Let them compete with each other instead.

Lastly, it is very important that the Contestant Manager not use this opportunity for sexual advances. The contestants have their hands full with the competition, and they need a helper and not a seducer. Sexual pressure can spoil the contest experience completely for contestants and generate the wrong kind of gossip for the promoters. Sexual neutrality should be the watchword here.

About Emcees

The emcees are in a position to manipulate the audience and judges in favor of their own favorite contestant. This can be done in a number of very subtle ways: emcees can use their voices to emphasize a particular contestant's name; the emcees can give their favorite or the audience's apparent favorite contestant more time on the stage than the other contestants are allowed; they can mispronounce a contestant's name; the emcees can indicate through body language that they find one contestant particularly hot or attractive. Emcees who have to make up questions can ask easy or interesting questions of their favorite. These and a host of other practices can indicate favoritism.

This kind of behavior is grossly unfair to the other competitors and should not be tolerated. However, once the show is underway, it is often too late to correct the problem because of production distractions. The Producer/Director should carefully remind the emcees not to tease, harass or otherwise make fun at any contestant's expense. Being out there on stage can be tough enough all by itself without having to deal with an insecure emcee's off-the-cuff remarks. A good emcee can make a contest really fun. S/he should have enough imagination to be entertaining without creating more problems for the contestants themselves.

Occasionally, this practice can be corrected during an intermission or when the judges are willing to stop the show to complain, but by then, the damage already has been done to certain contestants and can not be undone. Often, members of the production team can inadvertently show their own favoritism and this should be avoided through advance warnings to all concerned. Emcees who persist in either harassing contestants or showing favoritism do not show good sportsmanship and thereby forfeit the right to help at contests. Period.

The emcees should be told that they are expected to control the audience in favor of all the contestants equally. Audiences sometimes get rowdy during a show. Catcalls, booing and the like should be opposed by the emcees in the name of good sportsmanship. Some judges have stopped shows when the audience was so noisy that contestant's remarks could not be heard even at the judge's table. This makes the emcee look weak and unprofessional, and encourages the audience to conclude that titleholders are egotripping.

The emcees must understand how to control an audience and be willing to be firm. A good understanding of group psychology is almost an essential here. A contest is a kind of controlled party as far as the emcee and audience is concerned. But the one part of all good contests that requires the emcee to manage an audience most carefully is that part where the contestants must give a short speech.

Whereas it can make for a good time to engage in banter with contestants to help put them at ease during the other parts of the competition, this practice is definitely not advised during the contestants' speaking portion of the competition. Banter before each speech requires the audience to move from a party mood to a serious mood every few minutes—much too demanding a task for any audience already enjoying itself. For this reason, at the international shows, once the speech portion of the competition has begun, the emcees first quiet the audience, but thereafter, the emcees do not interact with the contestants except to introduce them by name and number. In this way, the audience can keep its concentration and quiet while the judges render their scores. Also, banter between speeches breaks a contestant's concentration on the speech—usually the toughest part of the event for most contestants and the one that the judges usually pay closest attention to.

The entire production team must get behind each and every contestant and support them through the contest. Only in this way do people in the contestant pool get the message that it is safe to take the risks that are always associated with competition.

Promoters, ignore this at your peril! Judges can and will stop a show that looks unfair in these ways. Our community is not served by this kind of behavior.

Judges, Judging, and Scoring

How you want to handle the judging of your contest depends mostly on how seriously you want the contestants and the audience to take your event. Sometimes, if the contest is strictly a "just for fun" event, you can let audience applause select the winner. I have seen this work well in a weekly bar contest. The winner is chosen by audience applause and goes on his or her way, never to be seen again.

If, on the other hand, you want to provide your community with some leadership, and/or send your winner on to bigger and (hopefully) better things, then you will want to have a winner selected who can command some respect. For this to happen, you will have to rely on experienced judges to choose the contestant who has the best chance at a more influential title.

When this is your goal, you can usually achieve the desired result by selecting celebrities, including popular titleholders, to be your judges. Having them there and publicizing their participation in advance will generate a bigger crowd, increase the chances of picking a winner who can do well in bigger contests, and signal to the audience that the title is also about leadership and community responsibility, which add up to leather prestige. This usually means more effectiveness in fundraising for charity, and it works.

If your contest is to be taken seriously by the community, it is important that your judging panel also have non-titleholders as well. Some good choices are: a representative from the charity that money will be given to if the representative is a leather person; officers of leather/levi clubs or organizations; owners of stores that cater to us if they are leather folks; writers, editors or publishers of leather-oriented publications; and people with a history of fundraising or political activity in the leather community. More and more often these days, it is possible to find people with several of the above qualifications.

Also, it is a good idea to have at least a few judges on your panel from outside your immediate locality. These are less likely to be acquainted with your contestants. This reduces the possibility of charges about a "rigged" contest.

In some localities, there is a trend to include opposite gender judges on the judging panel. This is not a bad idea; however, it is important to audiences that men's contests be judged primarily by men, and vice versa for women's contests. Also, in many places, the outgoing titleholder is customarily included on the judging panel. This person usually has a big investment in the selection of his/her successor, and therefore takes judging responsibilities very seriously. This custom prevails in all the major national and international shows.

How Many Judges?

For a monthly contest, the winners of which may go on to compete with each other for an annual bar title, three or four judges are plenty. For a bar title, five judges is customary: fewer than this and scoring can get sticky (unless the judges are all heavyweight titleholders, which is rare for a bar contest).

For a state or regional contest, five judges are the minimum, and seven or eight judges are the most that is practical. Seven is most common and quite workable. National and international events are usually judged by seven to nine judges, plus an alternate in case one should be disqualified, become ill, or drop out for some reason.

In general, no more than half of your judging panel should be composed of titleholders, lest you create the impression in the community that titleholders are only good for making jobs for themselves. You can be flexible about this, depending on who is available or already may be planning to attend.

These days, the experienced national level judges will often notify promoters when they are going to be attending and volunteer to fill out a judging panel. At popular events, the panel may end up titleholder-"heavy" as a result. This is not a bad thing, but it is less than ideal.

You can also avoid the charge that the results are all political because titleholders all know each other. Many in the leather community have the mistaken notion that titleholders only hang out or play with each other. Only titleholders know how untrue that is. Also, by having non-titled people judging, you give them another way to participate in leather community life. Vendors like to be seen as giving to the community as well as taking; having them on your judging panel helps fulfill that need.

Don't wait until the last minute to line up your judging panel. It looks bad to the audience if you are running around at the eleventh hour trying to scare up a qualified judge. Also, judging a contest requires the judges to get into a certain frame of mind to do the job, and this is hard to do at the last minute.

Special Issues Regarding Judges' Ethics

Your winner and new titleholder is not helped when there are suspicions about the integrity of the judging process. In fact, all your best efforts and the efforts of your staff can be instantly erased when people develop suspicions about the scoring outcome. It is, therefore, important that you take steps to prevent this from happening to yourself and your winner, contestants, judges and community. Everybody loses when these problems happen.

Here are some suggestions that can help:

- A judge should be willing to consider disqualifying him or her self or being disqualified if there has been too close a personal relationship with any contestant. (You decide what "too close" means.) The wisest course is for the judge to halt the judging process as soon as s/he becomes aware that this situation exists, explain the circumstances of the relationship to the other judges and they could decide.

  The judge in question could trade places with the alternate judge and continue. Another possibility is that the judge could disqualify him/herself only for scoring that particular contestant, but this decision must be made carefully. Another possibility is that the judge calls the matter to everyone's attention (in a private meeting) and a decision is made to proceed. At least the matter was brought out into the open and others were consulted. Consider informing all the contestants in a group when something like this happens, and you can nip gossip in the bud.

In most situations where this has come up, the judge in question did not disqualify. S/he either asked the contestant at issue very tough questions to dispel any air of favoritism, or the judge remained silent and the other judges questioned the contestant extra closely.

Certainly, judges should not create this situation for themselves by playing with or spending private time with any contestant at any time immediately prior to the selection of the winner.

For this reason, promoters should require their contestants and judges to wear their identification badges every time and every place they are likely to encounter each other. This minimizes the risk that a visiting titleholder or other judge might arrive in town for the event, go out, pick up a contestant as a trick by accident, and only then discover later that it was a contestant.

- Use a modified olympic scoring system to neutralize any possible favoritism. (See Judging below for an explanation of this system.)

- Arrange for the services of an outsider accountant to oversee the score tabulation and announce this fact before tallying begins. This can easily be the treasurer for the charity to benefit when the contest is a fundraiser.

- Producers should distance themselves from the tally process to avoid charges of tampering. Announce that the senior titleholder present, an outsider accountant, and some other independent person will be responsible for the tally of the scores unless one of these people is intimately involved with one of the contestants.

When the senior titleholder there is IML, IMsL, or Mr.

Drummer, and is personally involved in the tally process, there is the presumption that the result is above suspicion because that person's integrity is usually less in question than anyone else's. Quite often, the senior titleholder present serves as the head judge so such an announcement does not surprise either audience or contestants. It should reassure them.

- Arrange for three people who are not associated with each other or any contestant to be responsible for tallying the scores in a private place. If necessary, tactfully remind the tally people not to get loaded so that they don't jeopardize the process. Replace them if there is a perception that they are incapable.

- Require that the collected judges' score sheets never be left in any one person's hands during the entire contest once judges have submitted their sheets for tallying. If, for example, scores from afternoon prejudging must be held by one person until the night portion of the contest, it is very wise to seal the score sheets in an envelope in front of the entire judging panel and ask the head judge to sign his/her name across the flap. Only then is it safe for one person to hold the sheets until later.

- Double check all addition. That means that each contestant's overall score is re-calculated until the same sum is achieved twice. Re-assign the scoring jobs to different members of the tally panel for the re-calculation.

- Withhold the results from the judges after the tally is complete so that they themselves do not know who the winners are. Make them wait for the announcements like everybody else.

- Consider making the tally of total scores available to the contestants, judges, and contestant sponsors so that all can see how each contestant placed. This is especially helpful to contestants who are serious about wanting to hold a title. It reveals where their weak areas are so they can better prepare for next time.

- Explain to the audience how the Interview segment works. This way, they can conclude that if the hottest or prettiest contestant (who may be the crowd favorite) doesn't win, it may be because s/he blew the pre-judging portion of the contest.

- Promoters of contests should tell judges exactly what is being looked for in a winner. This can be done in a preliminary meeting with the judges or with a written handout provided to the judges so that they can study it. Otherwise, the promotor leaves it up to the judges to guess about what is desired.

Personal Arrangements for Judges (or Proper Care and Feeding of Judges)

Judging a contest can be a thankless task. It requires the judges to pay attention to the contestants in a very critical way and to pay particular attention to things that the ordinary contest goer might not even notice or care about.

Judges sometimes have to travel long distances, often at their own expense, just to have great seats for a contest which they don't get to enjoy in the same way that others can. Also, it is not fun to assign a low score to a contestant who is trying hard to win. While it is true that judges choose the winners, they also choose the losers, and there is no joy in that task.

For these and other reasons having to do with simple courtesy, it is important to make the judges' job as easy as possible. That way, you, the promoter, are more likely to get the judges' best efforts, which is what you want. Additionally, it is only fair to the contestants, without whom there would be no contest, to not distract the judges from their task with annoyance and inconvenience. Finally, your reputation sticks with judges as well as contestants: If you want to draw quality judges next year, treat this year's panel well. Here are some tips:

- Assign someone to be in charge of seeing to the judges' needs. This person should be a diplomat because some judges have large scale egos that can be a problem. S/he should also have the necessary authority to implement decisions affecting the treatment of the judges. S/he needs to be plugged into the production team at a high enough level to make his/her voice heard by key personnel.

- It is wise for both visiting and local judges to receive a schedule of the entire weekend event as soon as possible (preferably a week before the event) so they know where they are supposed to be and when. Don't hesitate to disqualify judges who show up more than 15 minutes late. This is another good reason to have an alternate judge on the panel.

  An advance schedule helps judges plan what free time they may have. Judges should not have to discover at the last minute that a contest official is expecting them someplace they had not prepared for, and that they must now cancel a lunch date with an old friend to which they were looking forward.

  Special Note: If you have one particular person on your judging panel who you have scheduled very heavily to make many appearances in connection with your event, you should consider the merits of assigning or at least offering a "handler" to help that celebrity. This handler can be responsible for transportation and can insure that your star is always on time, every time. This handler usually becomes a kind of personal secretary for the celebrity and introduces him/her to your VIPs at events and takes care of minor details in connection with the celebrity's appearances.

- Judges need to see their judging schedule during the event so that they know exactly when they are expected to observe the contestants and render a score during the contest. Having to guess about this makes judges anxious and angry. "Were we supposed to give a score just then?" is an unnerving question to hear at the judge's table.

  Any judge can and should stop the contest in it's tracks if he can't figure out what he is supposed to do about scoring and when.

This sort of interruption creates the impression that promoters are disorganized, and the audience can quickly lose its respect for a contest. These frustrations can cause a judge to think twice before accepting another invitation to judge.

Scoring is a bit less of a problem for the experienced judge, but instructions must be written for the judge who has never done it before and may never do it again. The charity representative who has agreed to serve as a judge cannot be expected to know what to do with an unclear set of judging instructions. The vast majority of titleholders may only get to judge one or two contests ever, so don't assume that having a title equals having judging experience.

Have a meeting with the judges to get clear about all these things. Leave time for questions.

Judges are more likely to render an objective score if there is some assurance given to them that their specific scores will remain confidential—that their name will not be connected with their score.

- Judges can and often do make their own housing arrangements with friends in the city they are coming to for the contest. But sometimes they go to cities where they have no friends, and rely on the promoters (Judge Coordinator—usually an Assistant Director) to make arrangements for them.

  Before the judge arrives, s/he should know the name, address, and phone number of his/her hosts, and the name and phone number of the person responsible for his or her transportation to and from the host home and to and from the events where one is expected to serve as judge. If the judge rents a car, be sure that s/he is provided with a map that helps him/her go where they need to be. If a taxi is to be used, make all of this clear ahead of time. Please do not expect judges to pay for their own ground transportation.

  If you arrange for a judge's transportation from home to

event, tell your transport person not to leave the event without first checking with the judge to see if s/he needs to be taken somewhere. Judges: If someone gives you a ride somewhere, make some arrangement about departure plans.

- Please do not make judges sit through long rehearsals if the judges are not needed. The Producer/Director should step the judges through their own stage presentation until each judge knows what is expected, and then discharge them. If judges must be held for rehearsals, provide food and drink at no charge.

  It is very unwise to allow judges to observe any part of contestant rehearsal. Rehearsals are places where it should be safe for contestants to make a mistake and fuss with their presentation. Sometimes rehearsal reveals a weakness in the contestant's approach to a problem in a fantasy, for example. Judges should only be allowed to view the finished product.

- The Judge Coordinator should be sure to provide: ample and safe seating space with a good view of the stage area that is free from the prying eyes of the audience; adequate lighting to make scoring accurate and easy (cheap battery-operated lamps work fine, or you can supply each judge with a small pen light); clear instructions about when the judges must observe for scoring purposes; extra pencils; matches & ashtrays for smokers, and, importantly, a person or two to see to the needs of the judges during the contest (to get drinks, to get notes to the director, whatever). In some places, these helpers have sometimes been called, "judge slaves" and they provide folks who have the need to serve others with a rare opportunity to serve in a public setting. Any refreshments delivered to the judges' table should be complimentary.

- Remember to provide a private and quiet place where the scores can be tallied. An adding machine is essential, preferably one that makes a tape—a tape makes it easier to double-check addition.

- Nice, though not necessary, extras can include: free commemorative pins, T-shirts, posters, mugs and such; free refreshments during the event; and a thank you letter from the Producer a few days after the event. Boutonnieres are not necessary.

Scoring The Contestants

Interview vs. Prejudging—A Distinction With A Difference

"Prejudging" implies a preliminary elimination of contestants which is usually done to prevent having an unwieldy number of contestants in the contest, which can take up way too much time. Technically, a prejudging elimination could be based on almost anything the promoters decided on—appearance, standard questions, etc.

At this writing, there is one contest that consistently uses a true preliminary elimination called "Prejudging" to reduce the number of contestants who continue in the competition. That is the International Mr. Leather contest.

The method used to reduce the number of contestants to a predetermined number of finalists happens to be a private interview (described later) conducted in front of the entire judging panel. Typically, the finalists are announced near the beginning of the night portion of the contest.

The majority of contests do not conduct an elimination round of competition simply because there are not usually enough contestants to justify making a cut in their numbers. Where this is the case, the interview segment is not used to eliminate, but merely to determine the best person for the job as part of the overall scoring.

An "Interview" means just that, questioning by others. It may or may not be part of a preliminary elimination called Prejudging.

Because the ability to represent, lead, inspire, teach and motivate the leather community has become so important in the selection of winners these days, the interview segment of the leather contest has moved into a position of prominence during the scoring process. No longer are winners expected merely to look good and command visual attention; they are now expected to be knowledgeable about the lifestyle, have good communication skills, and have at least minimal political savvy.

Promoters who omit this judging category cannot expect their winners to be taken seriously or compete successfully at the bigger regional, national and international contests. Promoters at smaller local shows can prepare their winners to compete more effectively by giving their contestants experience with the interview segment at the local level. The importance of speaking and thinking abilities should be reflected in the categories that identify these skills, which means more points are awarded for interview and speech segments than for the "skin show" portions of the competitions.

What Is The Interview?

The Interview is usually the first category during which the contestants are officially evaluated. It is generally scheduled on the morning of the contest early enough to leave time for rehearsal in the afternoon, followed by the evening portion of the contest.

Typically, the judges assemble in a quiet, private room at a table equipped with good light, interview score sheets and pencils (not pens). Usually, a senior member of the production team is present, and the Interview may or may not be video taped. (Video tape can later be reviewed by the winner in preparation for further competition.)

Usually just before the Interview, the contestants draw their numbers to determine their order of competition. Numbers are handed out and usually worn when in the presence of judges including social situations, if judges are present. Usually, the head judge puts the contestant applications in contestant number order, reads it to the panel of judges and then asks the Contestant Manager to bring in contestant number one.

At some contests, the contestant applications are duplicated and assembled in a packet for each judge after they have been placed in contestant numbered order. This can be very helpful to the judges and eliminates the need for the applications to be read aloud, thus saving time. This also eliminates the necessity for judges to ask basic information questions, the answers to which are already on the application. Judges can then also be reading the application as they listen to the contestant and perhaps be stimulated to ask questions raised by information on the application.

It is customary for the contestants to stand at a position about 6 to 12 feet from the judges' table. Since most titleholder work is done while standing, it works best to interview the contestants standing. Then the judges, one at a time, ask the contestant any question the judge thinks will help all judges evaluate the contestant.

Not all judges will ask questions or are required to do so. Each contestant is usually asked at least two or three questions, but the questioning continues until all judges feel they have heard enough to render a score. When the judging panel falls silent, the head judge asks if there are more questions, and if not, the head judge excuses the contestant and the process is repeated until all contestants have been questioned.

As a rule, the judges do not confer about the contestants either between interviews or at any other time once the Interview segment has begun. If some judge has some very direct and compelling evidence of a contestant's unsuitability, the judge may choose to share that information with the judges only if that judge fears there is a chance the contestant may otherwise be a strong contender for the title. This is very rarely done and usually only when that judge is absolutely certain of some grave wrongdoing. (In one case, a judge knew that a contestant was soon headed for prison on a felony conviction and no appeal was planned. In another, a judge had overheard the contestant saying that his only reason for entering was his interest in the prize money. However, any such information is best shared in the form of a question during the interview/prejudging portion of the contest.)

The production team is wise to schedule about 8-12 minutes per contestant and allow time for the judges to take a break about every 8-10 contestants. After all have been questioned, the Contestant Manager brings all the contestants back into the room to stand in numerical order. This gives the judges a chance to adjust their scores if necessary. When score adjustments are complete, the contestants are excused and the head judge collects the score sheets, places them into a manilla envelope, signs his/her name across the flap in the presence of the other judges, and hands the envelope to the production team representative for safekeeping until the remainder of the judging has been completed during the public portion of the contest. Later, the envelope will only be opened in the presence of the other judges or tally persons.

Scoring for Smaller Contests

In a weekly or monthly contest where the audience chooses the winner by applause, the custom is to line all the contestants up on stage after their category presentations. Then the emcee reminds the audience to applaud for their favorite. Typically, the emcee declares it to be close between two contestants. The other contestants are asked to leave the stage with the "tied" contestants remaining. At this point, the audience is asked to applaud for only one contestant, and the tie is broken.

At city or state contests, usually there are four or five judges and the scores are totalled and the winner is chosen using the total aggregate scores of all five judges. See the Appendix for examples of scoring sheets.

Many local sponsors feel compelled to use the olympic system because they know it is used in the big shows. The hitch is that the system demands a minimum of seven judges in order to work at all. Many local contests use only five or sometimes four judges. If the olympic system were to be used in these, it would mean that each contestant's final score would be determined by only three (with five judges) or two (with four judges) judges' scores comprising the total. Doing this bases the result on a very small number of evaluations, and therefore is not fair.

For this reason, sponsors should not use the olympic scoring system with fewer than seven judges. Instead, where there are fewer than seven judges, sponsors should use the aggregate total without eliminating any of the judges' scores.

When using a simple total like this with no scores eliminated, the risk of favoritism increases dramatically. Fortunately, the trend in recent years is to use well-qualified judges whose reputation for integrity is usually beyond question.

The Olympic System

This system requires a minimum of seven judges to work well and is workable with up to 9 judges. More than 9 judges is unnecessary and cumbersome.

Basically, this scoring system is designed to eliminate favoritism from influencing the result just in case one or two judges is either playing favorites or is carrying a grudge against any contestant. There are two ways it can work: either by category or by totals. Let me explain.

When olympic scoring is used by category, (Interview, Jockstrap, Revealing Look, etc.) it means that the highest judge's score and lowest judge's score are thrown out in each judging category. When olympic scoring is used by total, this means that each judge's scores in all categories are first totaled for each contestant, and then the high judge and low judge have their totals eliminated.

Because most judges never participate in the tally process, many of them may not even be aware that there are two ways to apply the system. Since this is not something that judges tend to discuss, I am unaware that there is any consensus on which application of the olympic system is favored.

Although I have never calculated scores both ways to see if outcomes could have been different, I am sure that this might be possible. Again, it is a problem that comes from having no standard.

At present, the IML contest is scored by eliminating a judge's total score and not by each category. The elimination of judges' totals saves a step in the scoring process and is therefore faster when the tallying is done all at once after all the contestants have appeared. But when the tallying is done after each contest segment, and elimination is done by category, much time is saved that way as well.

The Mr. Drummer International contest is scored using elimination by category. This permits all the judges to participate in the judging of all contestants unlike the elimination by totals system.

When there are more than 10 contestants, any time savings system can be important. Either system has the capability of reducing the influence of possible favoritism or grudges. After discussing this issue with many promoters, it is clear that the consensus is to eliminate by category rather than by total, and I am persuaded that this practice is the more fair of the two.

This concludes the section on contest production. I hope that the reader will be left with a more complete awareness of just what can be involved when it comes to contest production.

WINNING THE LEATHER CONTEST

How To Prepare Yourself For Competition

First of all, it is important to be clear with yourself about why you want to enter a leather contest. Here are some questions that you need to answer before you proceed:

- Why do I want to enter?
- Do I just want to be on the stage for the experience?
- Do I want to place?
- Do I really want to win?
- Do I really want to win this time?
- Am I doing this for someone else? For whom and why?
- How do I really feel about the idea of a leather contest?
- How do I really feel about the leather lifestyle?
- How do I really feel about the SM lifestyle?
- Am I prepared not to win?
- If I win, do I think I will do a good job? Why?
- Do I have the time and money to do a good job with the title?
- Am I ready to win?
- If I am not ready to win, what needs doing so that I can get ready to win?
- If I win, am I prepared financially and otherwise to pursue the next highest title, and will I be expected to do so?

There are no wrong answers to these questions. There is only your own personal truth. It is okay if you just want to be on stage, have fun and don't care if you win. Contests are a good time and give contestants a chance to learn important things about themselves.

But unless you know these answers yourself, it is unlikely that you will be the winning contestant. If you do win without having answers to these questions, it will only be because none of the other contestants had answers either and the judges thought you were the best of an unaware bunch. But even though you may have won, your community will probably have lost something important. This section is designed to see that this does not happen anymore.

If, at any level, you want to compete effectively, read and study carefully what follows. If you don't care about doing well, then don't bother with the reading—just go out there and have a good time, and do it just for fun. And if so, don't let anybody give you any grief about your decision. There is no reason to feel guilty about entering a contest just for the sheer fun of it!

So, how to win? In short, the answer is, prepare, prepare, prepare!

Prepare what? Prepare everything! You have to get your mind ready, you have to get your spirit ready, you have to get your body ready, and you have to get your heart ready to win if that is what you expect to do. Unfortunately, the foregoing preparations are not yet quite enough to bag the title. There is that last hurdle, the stage, and that will be discussed shortly.

One useful way to look at competition is to think about what the judges are looking for. If you intend to win, you must convince the judges that you deserve their highest scores in all categories, and you must do it fast and smoothly.

Winners are usually selected by judges, not by audiences. From a judging point of view, the audience reaction is only important to the judges in that they want to learn whether a contestant understands how to present themselves in front of an audience or not.

Judges want the person who comes closest to being the perfect choice. Ideally, they want the winner to be very strong in these categories: body; intellect; knowledge of the leather/SM/fetish scene; appearance; friendliness, outgoing personality; self confidence; social skills; sense of humor; public speaking; political astuteness; good taste; sexual energy; good heart; and spiritual completeness.

Unfortunately, judges rarely have time to examine contestants on much more than body, brains, leather knowledge, public speaking, self-confidence, and social skills. At contests where an interview is not allowed, judges have even less to base their decision on.

This "Mr./Ms. Perfect" never turns up because this human doesn't exist and the judges know it. This means that judges must try to balance a contestant's strengths against his or her weaknesses. This is not a science; it is a difficult art. The contestant's job is to make it easy for the judges to choose him/her for the top spot.

Let's talk specifics.

About Your Body

The judges want a winner to whom the community can relate physically from the neck down. Usually, this means some muscle definition if you are a man, or one of the desirable female shapes if you are a woman, but it can mean simple presentability. Most contestants could look much better than they do simply by doing what their mothers told them to do: "stand up straight and don't slump your shoulders!"

Nevertheless, it remains true that the better shape you are in, the better your chances are in the "skin" categories. A good body won't hurt your chances unless you use it as a weapon against the audience. People (and judges are people) are turned off by an egomaniac who is clearly in love with him/herself. The "I'm hot and you're not" attitude is a quick ticket to last place. Except for the occasional fluke, muscles or shapeliness will no longer make up for bad attitude, no smarts or no social skills.

Since there is no one who is universally attractive, the judges tend to cut contestants more slack than you might imagine from the neck up. Many titleholders are rather average looking when you come right down to it. Still, good grooming is essential from the neck up, too.

In general, your body can be out of shape and you can still "place" in a contest, but it's tough to win unless your body has been tortured into something resembling perfection by today's standards of physical beauty. If you're out of shape, you can win if no other contestants look better and you have the other bases covered, and the shapely one does not have them covered.

Remember, many audiences have been shocked when winners were announced and best body or prettiest face didn't win. Often, the muscled beauties blew it in the interview or had some other deficiency that outweighed their looks.

In a sense, our bodies are the easiest thing about us to change in terms of preparations to win. It is much easier for most people to gain or lose 20 pounds than it is to overcome shyness or to learn how to be friendly or give a speech. In short, be in the best shape you can be, but whatever shape you are in, wear your body with pride.

Being Nearly Nude

At some point during competition, you will be wearing less in front of more people than perhaps at any other time in your life. Shyness will hurt you here. It may help you to think of your body as a gift that you have chosen to share in a limited way with many people for a few seconds—be generous, but not vulgar. Remember, a contest is not a porno movie—no one is expecting to see your privates or watch you bump and grind. If your contest has a fantasy segment, that might be the place to get bold with your sexual tastes. Otherwise, the judges want someone who is hot, but leaves us curious.

If you can, get tapes of contests and note what you like and don't like about how each contestant handles him/herself on stage. Then, practice your movement in front of a mirror or, better yet, video tape and study yourself critically. Watch how you move. Do you look comfortable? Excited? Confident? Happy? How do you hold your body? Do you move in an interesting way? Make the changes you think are indicated, and try it again and so forth until you are satisfied with how you look to yourself. The acid test is, "Would I give myself top scores if I were judging this show?" Until your answer is yes, you are not yet ready to win.

Your Stage Skills

A big problem about leather contests is that it takes one set of skills to win a contest, and a mostly different set of skills to do a good job with the title. Many fine men and women with great titleholder potential slip through the contest net and lose simply because they don't happen to have stage skills.

There is no way that you can read this and learn all there is to know about stage skills, but there are some tips here that should help you at least have an even chance with the other contestants who are stage savvy.

To illustrate the points that follow, you might want to consider viewing a copy of one of the IML, IMsL or Mr. Drummer International videos.

Judges want a winner who demonstrates that s/he can handle him/herself in front of an audience in an engaging way.

Having an interesting body will not help you if you don't know how to move in it, how to wear it, how to use it to create a powerful effect on the people who will watch it. Judges know that titleholders use their bodies and appearance to get people's attention. Like it or not, most leather audiences won't listen to you unless you can get and hold their attention. Your body and face are tools. The judges want to see if you understand this fact and how to use them as a means to exercise leadership and accomplish change in the community.

Judges want you to look and move in a gender-appropriate way, whatever that means to you. Be aware that they don't necessarily want you to be a caricature—like a Bluto or some stiff Macho Man or Queen of the Amazons. In a men's contest, judges may penalize you for behavior that is too delicate or feminine for most men's taste. It doesn't mean that you aren't a man—it means you aren't their man. The issues here are a bit different for women in leather contests because the women's community is more tolerant of variation than is the men's community.

You will not help yourself if the judges see that you are afraid of the audience or self-conscious in front of people. When you are on stage, try not to run from "the spotlight;" fill it up and bloom.

Consider the merits of varying your approach when on stage. If you always look angry when on stage, the judges and audience will conclude that you are an angry person and you will probably lose the contest. People want to know that you can be friendly and sexy at the same time—your chances at winning will probably be improved if you can get this across to them.

Your conduct on stage should be consistent with the message you are sending at that moment. For example, during the skinshow portions of the contest, let the audience and judges see you being sexy. When you speak, try to make your emotion fit your words. If you are angry about something, show it. If you are sad, let them see that. A well-planned leather contest will give you the chance to show your judges and audience a balanced sample of the kind of titleholder you are aspiring to be. As a contestant, your task is to take full advantage of those opportunities.

It can be very useful to spend some time pretending to be on a stage because that is where you will compete. Some contestants set up bright lights to stare at and to smile into. This gives you practice at being as blind as you will be when in front of an audience while you are pretending to be able see.

You are on a stage to be seen, not to see for yourself. Most contestants go out on stage, wince into the spot lights, discover that they can't see anything, suddenly start feeling like a bug under a microscope, look disappointed, and then somehow make their way to the safety of the wings. I call this the "startled deer" approach to being on stage, but it doesn't work. The judges want someone who knows how to appear before an audience and look at ease, whether s/he is or not.

What You Have To Say

Now, I want to discuss the parts of contest preparation that have to do with what comes out of your brain through your mouth when you speak, because no matter how good you may look these days, it is very hard to place, let alone win, if what you have to say is not well thought out and doesn't work.

Since most leather men and women don't usually go around talking about the leather lifestyle and the issues related to our sexualities, there is little chance to get practice at this. So if you want to win, you must give yourself practice doing just that. The name of the winning game is: Preparation and Preparation. If you don't prepare to win, you very likely won't. There are several correct ways to do this. Here is one that works well for most people.

The first part of the solution to the problem of preparation is to have something meaningful to say during and after the competition in the first place. Spend some time thinking about the leather community and form some opinions about it and where you would like to see it go. Think also about what you are troubled by in the leather world and what you love about it.

As part of this process, you may find it very useful to involve yourself actively in such leather/SM/fetish lifestyle advocacy groups such as the NLA or Gay Men's S/M Activists ("GMSMA"), and read their newsletters along with other national lifestyle publications where you will receive updated information on issues affecting us all, along with information about how the community is responding to these issues.

The next step is to outline some possible solutions to the problems you have identified. It's a good idea to use pen and paper if that will help you stay organized, and it usually does. Once you have done this, and this is very important, turn what you have written about problems and solutions into a series of written questions.

Put these questions on separate cards. Practice by reading your cards and answering out loud. I suggest you talk out loud to yourself often about these ideas because that gets you familiar with hearing yourself talk about these issues, and gives you practice at thinking "on your feet" about your subject. After you have done this in private, ask a friend to mix up the questions and quiz you as if s/he were a judge.

At first, s/he should only ask the questions that you have written down and already practiced with. Later, invite her/him to ask you other questions that might occur as the two of you go along. When you have done this enough to feel comfortable, invite a small group of supportive friends (5-8) over to help you prepare for the contest. Explain to them what you are doing, and distribute your cards to them and get them to ask you your questions. This will simulate speaking before the panel of judges that you will be facing during the competition. It is next to impossible to win these things without lots of support from those who care, and this is a good time to rely on your friends.

Concentrate on keeping your answers to at least two sentences, but no more than five ever. The trick is to be short and complete in your answers. The less time you take to answer your questions from the judges, the more questions they will have a chance to ask you. When the judges find your answers interesting and your presentation appealing, they will hold you for more questions.

This means that judges will get a more rounded picture of you.

Humor helps too, if you already know how to use it well. It can also take the edge off a tense interview session and show the judges that you are comfortable enough with yourself to not be threatened by whatever they may ask.

Judges will be expecting you to be able to think on your feet because they know that many strangers both in and outside the leather scene approach titleholders to ask about the lifestyle. Judges want you to be able to rise to this challenge. If you don't prove to them that you can do this, they will have a difficult time choosing you as the winner.

You don't have to be into SM, but you had better know plenty about it because it is usually associated with the leather lifestyle. Read books that explain it well. The best choices currently available are *Learning The Ropes - A Basic Guide to Safe and Fun S/M Lovemaking* by Race Bannon, *Leatherfolk* edited by Mark Thompson, and *The Lesbian S/M Safety Manual* edited by Pat Califia. Since so many are also familiar with them, you would be well advised to be at least conversant with *Urban Aboriginals* by Geoff Mains, and *The Leatherman's Handbook*, 2nd edition (revised) (not the fiction parts) by Larry Townsend. I also believe my book, *Ties That Bind: The SM/Leather/Fetish Erotic Style—Issues, Commentaries, and Advice*, would be helpful in learning about SM. These books explain the SM scene well enough and will at least help you be conversant with the issues. The judges know that you will be asked about the SM scene if you become the titleholder, so have some answers. These days, there are over 200 clubs and organizations in the U.S. and Canada (about half that number overseas) who will be happy to make this information available to you.

About Judging

In most contests, you are judged on what you have to say two times officially (usually) and one or more times un-officially (usually). Let me explain.

At most contests, there is social contact between the judges and the contestants. This is either organized in some kind of a "judges meet the contestants" situation like a cocktail party, or judges bump into contestants in the course of getting ready for the contest. Try to make contact with all the judges.

Contestants, don't kid yourselves. Most competent judges will notice how you handle yourself both on and off the stage. Pay attention to how you speak to judges in any situation as well as what you have to say. I am not suggesting that you lobby the judges as to your suitability for the title, but this is when the judges get a feel for your ability to socialize.

These are not good times to let them see you drunk, angry, arrogant, super scared, shy, seductive, or catty. And yes, more and more, judges watch you speak with others and make mental notes. These are the subtle points that don't show up on the score sheets in any category, but they can sometimes count plenty. These are the unofficial opportunities the judges have to judge contestants.

Officially, contests are usually arranged to provide the judges a chance to ask questions of the contestants privately at some point, often early on the day of the contest. This is called Prejudging or the Interview (see comments on the interview/prejudging segment in the previous production section). Each contestant is brought before the panel of judges, and they are allowed to ask any question they wish. You are not obligated to answer questions you don't wish to answer, but think carefully about declining any question. This process rarely lasts more than 7-10 minutes for each contestant, so you don't have a lot of time to put yourself across to the judges.

For the judges who didn't get a chance to meet you earlier, this may be their very first impression of you. First, they look at what you wear and how you carry yourself. Smile when appropriate and, at some point during the prejudging, try to look each one of the judges straight in the eye and hold their gaze for a moment, speaking directly to that judge. There is almost no chance that you will win if you can't smile and be friendly with people.

Your appearance should make it clear that you are really a leather/kinky person, but not be too far out. Most judges want to choose someone to whom the mainstream community can relate and not be turned off by. You will have to decide how to express your individuality visually, yet keep your connection to the mainstream. That is always the challenge of choosing what to wear during all judging segments.

Contestants tend to do better if they don't turn the contest into a fashion show. I suggest that you avoid Las Vegas-type get-ups. They may distract the judges from listening to what you have to say. I also suggest you wear only your own stuff even if it is new (some contests require this) because that's what you will be most comfortable in, and it is what you may be asked to wear in future appearances after winning. This doesn't mean that you shouldn't take risks with your attire, just be careful. Remember, when you win, you will have to represent all leatherfolks.

At many contests, judges get to read over your application in advance of prejudging, and they may select questions from your own application. Think of this when you fill it out. Sometimes judges ask questions about something you are wearing and what it means to you. You may be asked about how you came to be a leatherman or leatherwoman, how you have been of service to the leather community, or how you came to the decision to enter the contest. These days, there are often political questions about AIDS policy, women in leather, our relationship to the non-leather communities, the value of boycotts, forced outing, and so on. If you want to win, prepare!

Another chance judges will use to find out how you think and speak is when you give your speech during the public portion of the contest. The trend is to place a time limit on speeches, usually not more than three minutes (at IML it's 90 seconds). Generally, contestants are allowed to speak about anything they wish.

Speak in English if you are before an English speaking audience. If you want the judges to know that you speak some other language, mention that in the "special interests" part of the application. Don't say you speak a language if you don't. Many judges speak more than one language and you may be tested with an off-hand remark. I, myself, have caught contestants in this lie.

Sound systems can do strange things to your voice, especially in a very large room. Try not to speak too fast or your words may become garbled in the acoustics of the room. Pronounce your words clearly and try to use different ranges in your voice to emphasize the points you will make. Ask to use the microphone during rehearsal so you know how your voice will sound in the room and get a bit of practice hearing yourself in that space. Most successful competitors take the microphone out of its stand and move around a bit when speaking to hold the audience's visual attention—practice this way.

Although notes may be used, I don't suggest them because they will break your connection with the audience and you will probably ruin your chances to win if that happens. Judges know that titleholders get asked to speak with only a moment's warning, or often with none at all. Usually, judges will feel better about selecting you as the winner if you show them how comfortable you look speaking without notes. This means that you either make your speech "off the cuff," or you memorize something almost word-for-word, or you can memorize a short list of ideas you want to include and then make your speech up as you go along. I have seen various titleholders use any of these methods equally well, but whatever you choose, it will usually have to be delivered "blind" because you will probably be staring into a spotlight when you speak. I suggest that you smile when appropriate, and look into the spotlight as if you could see your audience perfectly. Practicing this at home is easy. Just shine a bright light in your face, stand, and deliver.

These days, in a few contests, questions are sometimes still written out in advance and the contestants are expected to answer them live, on stage, with maybe 10 to 15 seconds to think about the answer. Although this used to be a standard part of the Mr. Drummer contests, it has been dropped because it was unwieldy, time consuming, and unnecessary.

From my point of view, this is the most tricky situation for contestants to face because rehearsal and preparation for this is next to impossible. I have seen more contestants crash and burn here than in almost any other way.

If the question happens to be one that you have prepared for, then there is not usually too much trouble. If you can turn one of your prepared answers into the answer to the surprise question, then that can usually work out well also, but be sure to answer the question that has been asked.

The danger comes when the question is funny, but empty or irrelevant. For example, "What well known man is your idea of what sexy is all about?" is the kind of a question that can destroy an unwary contestant. This was an actual question in a real contest that hurt an otherwise strong contestant.

Other kinds of trouble questions are those that ask too broad a question. The contestant is asked to condense too much information into a short answer and often ends up fumbling around with too much data to organize quickly into a good answer. "Tell the audience what 'leather' means to you" is a typical example. You might as well be asked to describe the universe and give three examples.

My only advice on how to answer a silly, empty or too complex question is to think about it long enough to turn it into a meaningful question with how you answer it. In the above example, you might say something like "Lots of different things can be sexy to me; sometimes it is looks—Harrison Ford comes to mind. But sometimes it is bravery, and then I think of Nelson Mandella or Han Solo. Or perhaps it might be better to think in terms of wit and charm, and then I think of Michael Pereyra (a former IML titleholder) (unless he is judging that night). I would want a sexy man to embody all these traits. Sexiness is so much more than appearance," is an answer that might work in this situation.

When the question is just too broad to cope with, try to pick the part of the answer that is most meaningful to you and speak about that. For example, if confronted with the "what does leather mean to you" question, you might answer "Well, there are too many things to mention right now, but the part that means the most to me has to do with the way that leather is a bold statement about the willingness we have to be different and not to apologize about a part of us that is controversial, but central to our lives. It means we are unwilling to live in fear even though that means taking a risk." Judges would respect such an answer.

The third kind of tricky question asks you to take a position on an issue where the mainstream leather community itself is about equally divided. Usually you can tell when one of these has been asked because you get a sinking feeling in your gut. It's almost a sure sign that you must beware.

For example, "Do you think there should be a dress code in our leather bars?" My feeling is that it is usually best not to take a position in these controversies because that risks alienating those in the audience who take the opposite position, and you may hear them boo—not good for your confidence and it makes judges nervous. It is, I think, best to discuss briefly both sides of the issue and say, "Yes, this is a problem, and I don't know the answer." You will be respected as a diplomat with such an answer. If you do decide to take a position on a controversial issue, be certain that you have thought the issue through thoroughly and can make your case clearly and quickly for the judges.

Whatever the speaking situation, one last rule is an absolute must—speak up and articulate your words! The only nightmare worse for a judge than a contestant who has nothing to say is a contestant who has nothing to say and who can't be heard or understood. And a bitter frustration for judges is to face an otherwise stellar candidate who has a long history of community involvement, but who couldn't talk his or her way out of a paper bag.

If you have problems making your voice work, consult a speech therapist or a voice coach. Don't let your good words get lost in a mumble that could easily be corrected with a little professional help.

Fantasy Issues And Design

A fantasy is really a skit which often has an erotic theme. Having to perform a fantasy as part of a competition has special problems and the solutions require some careful thought. Usually, there is a three-to-six minute time limit imposed by the contest managers. Even three minutes on stage can feel like an eternity if you are not accustomed to performing, so this must be well planned.

You want people to understand your fantasy when they see it. Don't expect too much from your audience in terms of understanding complex symbolism. Some of those watching have never seen a fantasy before. These are the ones you should design your fantasy for, not in terms of content, but in terms of clarity.

Contestants are wise to remember that many people will want to see the details of the fantasy and it should be planned such that this will be possible. "Close work" such as knot tieing, piercing, and hot wax is usually impossible to see from the back row and runs the risk that you will lose your audience. People lying flat on the stage also cannot be seen. In some situations, the stage is below eye level. Make sure that all the action you want the audience and judges to see takes place above eye level or it will be lost on the audience. When the stage area is deep, try to plan the action more toward the audience so people can see it. Gestures should be "stage sized"—large enough to be seen and understood in the back of the room. Remember, many in the audience have come and paid good money specifically to see the fantasy performance. Stage it so that they can really see it.

Think about smoothness as the fantasy unfolds. A stage is not a playroom where you can take your time to solve technical problems as they come up. Rehearsals at home will often reveal staging problems that you won't want to solve on stage in front of an audience and the panel of judges.

Consider presenting a fantasy and not a reality. The audience needs to know that what they see is inside someone's head, and not just a peek in on a standard scene. Think about stage craft. Knots that will have to be untied during the presentation do not need to be really tied tightly. You would have to fumble to do the untying and the audience would see this.

Avoid using a cast of thousands. The contestant will get lost and the audience and judges want the contestant to be featured in the fantasy. When contestants wear hoods and such, we may not be able to figure out who is who.

When you are working out the blocking (who stands where on the stage), make sure that the audience, especially the judges, can see all that is going on—that we don't have to look around somebody to see what is going on behind the person in front. Judges do not appreciate having to strain to see what is happening, and may penalize contestants when it's time to dole out the points. Think in terms of displaying the action "side-to-side" rather than "front-to-back" on the stage.

If you are going to do anything requiring kinky technical skill on stage such as bondage, whipping and such, make very sure that you know what you are doing and play safely and smart. If the judges see you doing anything that is technically unsound you will likely suffer in the points department. In some contests, helpers have come off stage after a fantasy with numb wrists, unwanted bruises, unexpected cuts, and the like. Word gets out because unhappy people talk, including judges, other contestants, and helpers.

Animals are unwise to include in fantasies. The theater may have rules about them, they could be injured, get in the way, behave unpredictably during the performance, and so on.

If you need to use electricity on stage, make sure that your batteries are fresh or that the outlet you will use is working when you will need to use it. More than a few fantasies have crashed and burned for this mistake.

There are restrictions in many places about the use of fire on stages. Candles may be permissible on one stage, but not allowed on others. Flashpots can be very dangerous and spew hot materials in unpredictable ways—best to think of something else.

Try to design your fantasy such that nothing splatters on the stage. This makes trouble for the stage hands and you need them on your side. If the stage hands forget to pick up something you left behind, it may cause trouble for some other contestant. At one contest, a specially prepared bottle was broken over someone's head, and small pieces of glass were all over the stage; judges (who could see the glass) stopped the show for a clean-up. A broom had to be found, and the continuity of the event was interrupted.

Please, please, please don't throw things off the stage into the audience—most especially, not at the Judges! Nobody wants to be squirted with fake cum, catch a boot or clothes pins in the face, and the like. One contestant had his motorcycle on stage and started it up as the climax to his fantasy—accidentally in gear. It nearly flew off the stage and into the audience when he took his hand off the clutch to wave at the crowd.

The Producer/Director will need a script of the fantasy which includes music and light cues (see example in Appendix). Work your rehearsals out from the script so that the script is a "recipe" for the fantasy. Send a copy of the script and a copy of the tape of your music to the Producer/Director. Also included must be a map of the stage indicating what equipment is to be placed where, and a list of the equipment and props you plan to be using. Keep a copy of this list and use it when you pack and unpack your gear.

If you will need any special effects (smoke, mirrors, projection equipment, etc.) make arrangements to bring them along or to secure them in the city where the contest will take place in advance. The Producer/Director may not be able to provide exactly the lighting and other special effects you specify, especially if it is complex in any way—best to keep it simple and flexible.

Blue lights suggest night, death, depression; yellow lights suggest daylight, illness; red often represents anger, evil, danger, the underworld; green—illness or peace. Plan your lighting with care and to be consistent with the content of your fantasy. Pink light is good for flesh tones, and makes leather look like it is in daylight. Red light is very bad for videotaping.

If your taped musical accompaniment calls for silent parts, don't expect the sound person to stop and start your tape. Instead, record clean silences of the proper length directly on to the tape so the sound person just has to start the tape and play it straight through to the end. Don't trust your fantasy to a busy sound person who has many other things to worry about during your presentation.

Quite often, the sound reproduction equipment in theaters is either very good or very bad. For this reason, it is very wise to have the best quality sound you can manage on high quality tape.

Voice-over has been used in fantasies and has been sometimes very good and sometimes poor. It can be just one more element to be concerned about. If you insist on it, it should be fairly short and professionally produced. If the voice-over is a first person narrative and tells something about what is happening in your head, it should be in your own voice and carefully recorded so as to minimize echo. Remember to speak slowly and very clearly. Poor voice-over will lose the judges and audience fast.

Try to let your actions in the fantasy speak for themselves. If you have to explain too much using taped voice-over, it probably means that you haven't found a way to explain your fantasy with actions. Another problem with voice-over is that the sound reproduction quality, if poor, can cause the audience and judges to conclude that the whole fantasy is substandard.

Have your music tape cued up for the sound person with about five seconds of silence at the very start of the tape. Make sure your contestant number is directly on the tape cassette and also on the box it comes in. Submit only one tape. Arrive with one or two spare tapes just in case one gets lost.

When your turn comes to perform, get set up completely first (usually, the stage will be dark for set-up), then signal the stage manager or whomever is responsible for cuing the sound person, and off you go!

Leave nothing to chance. Remember Murphy's Law: If something can go wrong, it will.

The Winning Edge

If you want to arrive at the big international contests with all the aces in your hand, you will have to do some extra homework. It can help your image with the judges if they know that you already have a history of community service that has been public. You can accomplish this in a number of ways.

Writing articles and having them published in the major publications along with your photograph can help here. Appearing at community events as a leather person and helping the event promoters accomplish their goals is another way to do this. Offering your services to clubs and organizations with respect to leather/SM related seminars, demonstrations and such also shows the judges that you are committed and involved.

These accomplishments are only useful if you remember to mention them during the prejudging phase of the competition. Doing so can give you an edge over the contestants who have done none of these things. Generally, it is unwise to present your press kit to the judges unless they ask for one. Plan ahead, and rehearse your stage presentations until you've got it cold.

Some Tips About Competition In General

- Get some practice using a microphone, including raising and lowering it and removing it from its stand.

- Get rest the day and night before the show so you don't look tired.

- Study carefully any printed material you get from the promoters.
- Wear stuff that is really "you".
- Don't say things you don't believe in. (Don't lie!)
- If you don't know the answer, say so.
- Watch your mouth; people talk.
- Eat some honey one hour before the event for energy.
- If you smoke, don't chain smoke.
- Don't let your breath stink when you meet people.
- Cologne or after shave can be offensive.
- Use common sense.
- If this scene is all a joke to you, don't play to win. It just wastes everyone's time.
- Bright stage lighting makes pale people look like chalk; consider getting a tan—you will almost always look better under the lights.
- Remember to smile. If you always look angry or sad, you will lose for sure.
- If you are a bottom, be a bottom. Don't pretend to be a top. If you are a switch, you don't have to hide that either. Whatever you are, present yourself with the courage of your convictions!
- When you speak, do so "from the heart."

Remember, just because someone is your sponsor in the contest, that does not mean that they own you if you win. You have to follow your own destiny and not always step to the tune that your sponsor may have in mind. Once you win, it is important not to become the political lackey of your sponsor or you will risk losing your credibility. Be careful what you promise in advance.

By the same token, when a sponsor has gone the distance for you, whether or not you will continue to need his/her support, it is important to forge a close working relationship with such a person as equals or as partners in a process, if this is possible. Sponsors are people too, and they need the same strokes as contestants. Be sure to mention your sponsor publicly from the stage if the opportunity presents itself and think about your sponsor's needs for publicity when you are out and about.

If you leave your sponsor with a bad taste in his/her mouth, s/he may be reluctant to sponsor any contestant ever again, and you would have injured a community resource.

Unfortunately, the person or persons who sponsor you in the contest might or might not necessarily be the best people qualified to coach you in your preparations to win in a bigger competition. Talk to other titleholders or judges who are not judging the contest you want to enter for competition tips, but don't try to change your well worked out strategy at the last minute. It could throw you off balance during your presentations.

My point in spelling all this out is to stress the need to have your wits about you all during competition. The advantage of serious preparation if you want to win is that once you have done so, you can face the judges and the other competitors with much more confidence than you would otherwise have. It will show, and if you want the job, you will have to work to prove that to the judges who are expecting more and more from contestants than ever before. And that is because they realize that titleholders have more responsibility than at any other time in the history of our lifestyle.

Lastly, remember to have fun with all this. Otherwise, all the effort will never be worthwhile.

JUDGING METHODS AND ISSUES

Moving into the '90s, it is clear that the quality of contestants in general has been improving. As the leather/SM/fetish lifestyle gains more and more acceptability among its own practitioners, we see that a different calibre of person is now stepping forward to serve by holding title.

This fact makes judging an increasingly complicated job as we have more and more good competitors and (often) less and less time to make our evaluations. So to select the best person for the titles, it is important that we sharpen our skills when we sit down to look them over and choose a winner.

At this writing, there are about forty really well-qualified and experienced judges nationwide who can do the job and do it well. In time, more will join this group as the pool of experienced judging people grows. What follows is a series of ideas designed to help the local, less experienced judges choose the best person to hold title. These ideas might also serve to refresh the thinking of those who judge the larger regional, national, and international events as well.

When you are tapped to judge a contest, hopefully you will have at least one week before the event to collect your thoughts about the job. The best place to start the process of preparation to judge is in private with yourself. It can be very useful to spend some time thinking, and maybe taking some notes, about the needs of your community. This can include some ideas about what you think a titleholder might be able to do to improve the quality of life on the local scene.

Since there is not one single leather community, the job of holding title will look different from city to city. The needs of each locality are unique, and therefore require a specialized approach to get the job done. Furthermore, as communities develop, the job of holding title evolves with it. The right person for the job five years ago might not be first choice in today's climate.

For example, the more sophisticated a leather community becomes, the more likely it is to develop increasingly complex political problems. In one place, leather bar owners may not be speaking to each other. In another, there may be lifestyle oriented clubs or organizations that are "at war" with each other. Somewhere else, there may be an influential, but irresponsible, person who is the problem. Such difficulties don't help our community grow and flourish. Titleholders can be useful in these situations if they display a sensitivity to politics and are neutral enough to facilitate communication between factions.

In a way, a title is a job description that is particular for the community that the title is in. When judges don't consider the local situation, they run the risk of missing a great opportunity to perform a healing function in their area. By taking some time to think these issues through, a judge will be better prepared to tailor the titleholder job to the community situation at hand by selecting the contestant who best displays the desired skills.

Each judge is actually a kind of appointed "elector" who chooses titleholders on behalf of the community that is to be served by the titled person. This viewpoint will help you keep your task in perspective. For the most part, you have probably been asked to judge because the contest promoters were of the opinion that you understand your community well enough to know what the issues are.

The Judging Sequence

Judges will be expected to score contestants usually three or four times. The typical order is as follows —

First Appearance: Prejudging eliminations or Interview—usually on the afternoon of the contest. See description of the process in the previous Production and Competition sections.

Second Appearance: At the evening portion of the contest—usually in "casual" wear. The contestants are presented to the audience and some of their biography is read at that time.

Third Appearance: This is the jockstrap or skinshow portion. Contestants wear revealing attire, are presented to the audience as more of their biography is read.

Fantasy is performed. (Many contests do not use fantasies. For example, Mr./Ms. NLA does not, but Mr. Drummer and IMsL do.)

Questions are read from cards to contestants who answer "on the spot." (Not used often.)

Last Appearance: "Full leather" or "leather image" and a short speech is made—usually 90 seconds to three minutes.

Each of these appearances is designed to reveal both the strengths and weaknesses of contestants under different conditions. Let me explain.

The Interview (May Also Be An Elimination)

The Interview is the judges' chance to get an inward look at the contestants—to see their insides. Judges may ask any questions they like to "take the measure" of the candidate for the title job. This setting also lets judges see how the contestant handles him/herself when dealing with small groups and to determine each contestant's values, accomplishments, and vision for the community.

Each judge should take some time to decide what s/he thinks are the most important qualities in a titleholder and craft questions designed to assess these qualities. This is not play time. The contestants know it and may have prepared themselves very well for this appearance.

When the contestant seems well-prepared, it is a good idea to ask questions that will reveal the "human-ness," or the "heart" of the contestant. With well-prepared contestants, the real trick is to get behind any facade the contestant may be offering to the judges. This is not easy, but it is worth the effort.

This can also be a good time to find out how well informed the contestant is about the community s/he wants to represent.

Questions that might serve these purposes include —

- Why do you want this title?
- What will you do with it that is new and different?
- What do you see as the function and purpose of holding title?
- What problems are unique to this community, and what solutions to them would you implement?
- Tell us about your history in the community.

- Are you into the SM scene? In what way?
- What do the words, "Safe, Sane and Consensual" mean?
- What is a "safe word?"

To get at deeper issues:

- Who is Robert Mapplethorpe and why is he important?
- What are you most afraid of?
- Do leathermen and drag queens have anything in common or not? If so, what? If not, why not?
- Should leather bars have dress codes? If so, why? If not, why not?
- Should women be allowed in men's bars and vice versa?
- What do you think about "outing?"
- If you had to make two reading recommendations for a person interested in the SM/leather scene, what would they be?
- Should leather folks be out to their families?
- What ideas do you have about supporting racial minorities in their bid for acceptance in the leather scene?
- Should titleholders be seen in "play" settings playing?
- What should be done about titleholders who get drunk and abusive in bars?
- Do you color your hair? Why?
- What do you love most about the leather scene?

Clearly, questions like these can get into the issues quickly and reveal how a contestant thinks about the scene and what his/her relationship to it is. There is nothing unfair in thinking about your questions in advance. The contestants who want to win have prepared themselves, so why shouldn't you? If the other judges are not asking the questions you want answers to, ask them yourself! Just as you are allowed to ask any question, the contestants have the right to refuse to answer if they feel your question is improper.

Like it or not, the leather community has our fair share of shady characters. Unfortunately, from time to time, just such a shady character will enter a contest, and it is the judges' responsibility to see that none of these become titleholders.

Since most contest managers/promoters do not allow the

judges to consult, judges who have inside information that might influence the judging outcome negatively can, if they wish, bring this information to the attention of the other judges by asking a question. So you might hear questions like, "I have heard that you are being sent to prison in two months. Is this true," or "Complaints have circulated in the community about your business practices in connection with your mail order business. Would you care to comment?"

Judges who ask such questions risk the possibility that they will be accused of character assassination which is why it is so important for contestants to understand that any question may be asked during the interview segment of the contest. For this reason, it is doubly important that the judges bind themselves to a strict code of confidentiality with respect to the contestants' replies to questions. Remember, too, that contestants can always refuse to answer your questions.

When judging contestants not from North America, be mindful that AIDS related activities are not as well developed in other countries as is the case here. In countries where socialized medicine is the rule, there has been much less pressure on the community to provide money for services since they are paid for by the state. Also remember that sex education programs aimed at AIDS prevention are generally much better developed in most European countries than here.

In short, don't expect the same level of community action in foreign contestants that you may have come to expect from American competitors. The political and social problems that we face in the U.S. are not necessarily the ones faced by those from other countries. Questions relevant for U.S. contestants might not be appropriate for contestants from other countries.

The Casual Wear Walk On

How a contestant behaves in the privacy of the Interview segment may be very different from their manner on stage in front of an audience, and this will usually be your first look at this aspect of the competitors. Notice what s/he has chosen to wear. Is it appropriate? Is it believable? Is this a leather man/woman?

Titleholders will have to present themselves on stages many

times during their tenure. Keep your eyes open for stage skills. Who is comfortable and who is not? Body language can tell a great deal about a competitor. Look for signs of security and confidence. Are they having a good time?

Some judges prefer to keep the impressions gathered during prejudging in mind when evaluating contestants on stage during the evening portion of the contest, and others start with a clean slate for each judging category. Follow your own intuition about this, but keep your eye on the objective—to choose the best person. Remember, most titleholders don't do their job while wearing either jockstrap/skinshow type stuff nor while wearing "full leather/leather image" type wear; they dress in a more casual style.

Jockstrap/Skinshow

This is your chance to pick what you feel is the most appealing body on the stage in order of preference. The first issue that comes up here is how much sexual energy is the contestant able to project without being downright vulgar. A contest is not a porno movie, remember.

I find that most judges let this score come directly from their groin area and try to keep their heads out of it when possible. If you must evaluate this part with your head, think about how well the contestant moves inside his/her body and how much pride they have in it. Most contestants are at least a little exhibitionistic. See if it comes across.

Judging is hard work. Judges are human, too, and sometimes have to deal with their own personal preferences in the process of judging a contest. For example, some gay men have had only limited involvement with lesbians. Maybe, "If I were a straight man or a lesbian, which of these women would I lust for?" might help some gay male judges evaluate contestants in a women's contest. Some judges who never prefer black men or women try to evaluate them as if the contestant were white or vice versa as the case may be. If you never go out with tall people, it may be useful to see him/her as "just right" in the height department. Some judges try to neutralize what may be their own prejudices in this way. Think about it.

The Fantasy

Judging fantasies can be hell. As often as not, it is like comparing a Ferrari, a piece of cheesecake, a Bach cantata and a sunset—each to the other. Usually, the best way around this is not to compare them at all, but rather to evaluate each one on its own merits.

Here are some questions that can provide some useful guidelines for assigning a score: Does the fantasy "work?" Do I understand it? Does it stir anything in me? Does it come off smoothly? Is it a fantasy? Is it safely executed? Is it creative? Does it grab me somehow (hot, funny, thought-provoking, moving)?

Depending on the space allowed on judging forms, one trick is to assign a temporary score and then go back to change it after you have seen all the fantasies. The problem with this is that there are sometimes so many fantasies to look at that you can easily forget who did what. When fantasies are done well, they can draw you into them such that you can forget the others. When this happens with several of them, these could generally be the candidates for your highest scores.

The "Pop" Question

In a very few contests where this category is still used, the contestants (and sometimes the judges, too) are asked to fill out one or two index cards in advance, with questions written down on them. Next, a producer or head judge (hopefully) reads through them beforehand to eliminate duplications as well as inane, stupid, hurtful and illegible or unintelligible questions.

After the cards are mixed up, the contestant will be asked to draw a question on stage. When this is done correctly, the contestant selects a card, reads the question silently to her/himself and hands it to the emcee, who then reads it aloud to the audience over the microphone which gives the contestant a moment to prepare an answer. The emcee hands over the microphone and the contestant answers or responds.

From my point of view, this can be the most dangerous moment during competition for the contestants. The question can be stupid, too broad, or poorly written—problems which the contestant must try to overcome with his/her answer, and this must be done instantaneously and before a live audience. There is almost no chance to rehearse for this situation. Because of its unpredictability, most promoters do not give this category many possible points to earn. Yet, it must be scored.

Judges I have spoken with about this use different methods to assign points here. Generally, if the question is straightforward, relevant and not too broad, judges expect the contestant to respond with a really good and complete answer. In this situation, the contestants often get off easily because they can sometimes use one of their prepared answers for such a question. In some ways, it takes more skill to turn a dumb question into a good one with how it is answered. A contestant who draws an empty question is at the judge's mercy.

Full Leather And Speech

Again, this segment is about how the contestants look and what they say, as well as how they say it. Most judges tend to look for ease of delivery. Is this somebody who can speak effectively to an audience or not? Are the ideas sound? Is the reasoning clear? Is the voice one that commands attention and makes us want to listen? Do these words make sense coming out of this particular man or woman (has somebody else written the speech for him/her?). Does this language fit with what we already know about this contestant? Is this contestant saying anything new?

It is the emcee's job to quiet the audience before the speech segment of the contest begins, and to intervene whenever the audience gets too loud as the speech segment continues. However, if the emcee is unable or unwilling to quiet the audience, you, as a judge, have the right to complain first to the promoters. If the audience is still noisy, you can stop the show and speak earnestly to the audience or invite the noisy ones to step elsewhere until this part of the show is over. Judges may also have to protect the contestants during the competition from an unruly audience. Though difficult, this intervention is very important if the community is to have the best contestant chosen as its servant.

Scoring Tips And Ideas

Some judges find it useful to assign a score and a make a plus (+) or a minus (-) sign to the side when they think they might want to make adjustments later. That way, if they want to favor one competitor over another, they have given themselves some guidelines with which to adjust scores up or down.

Another device used during the evaluation process is to mentally assign all contestants a score in the exact middle of the point range just for walking through the contest. As their presentation unfolds, you can adjust up or down depending on how well you like or don't like what you see, hear and feel. To give an example from another part of life, I know people who, when dining out, start the waiter or waitress with a 15% tip the minute they sit down and adjust it during the meal silently in their heads. This scoring idea works the same way.

Most judges know that contestants are usually on their best behavior during the formal judging presentations. Some contestants are very skilled in their presentation of a facade at these times.

One possible way around this is to observe your strong candidates for high scores closely during the informal get-togethers that have become a part of most contests, and keep your impressions in mind during the judging. Good times to consider doing this are after the Interview but before the night portion of the contest.

Try to use pencil to do your scoring so that you can change your scores as your impressions of contestants change. Make certain that you know exactly when you are expected to render a score. If you are unclear about this, ask the head judge.

An unprofessional emcee or a missed sound or light cue can throw a contestant off badly. Some hostile, scared or inexperienced emcees delight in having fun at a particular contestant's expense. Most judges try to ignore this sort of behavior or, in some cases actually reward that contestant with a higher score for valor under fire. Other emcees have been known to emphasize their introductions of contestants to indicate who their favorite is. Judges may wish to ignore this and/or complain to the promoter if it persists.

In assigning your scores, use all the information about each contestant that you have at your disposal. Beware of gossip because it may not be true. Above all, trust your feelings. To do so, you must first be in touch with them. Alcohol and drugs make that difficult if not impossible to do, so think about your job responsibility before you order that next drink. You make your choices on behalf of the community when you are serving as a judge and everyone connected with the contest deserves the best that is in you for the few hours that you will spend judging.

Judging Etiquette

Usually, as a courtesy, the senior titleholder judge is chosen as the head judge by the promoters. However, the senior titleholder present may not have the experience to do the job correctly. In this circumstance, the promoters will do well to select the most experienced person available on the judging panel who will accept the job. Most inexperienced titleholder judges will be relieved when this happens.

Sometimes, the promoters and the other judges will look to the head judge for leadership during the judging process. Once the judging process has begun, if you, as a judge, have questions or concerns, it is a courtesy to voice them to the head judge and let her/him deal with the promoters on the matter. If the head judge does not resolve the matter to your satisfaction, then feel free to discuss the issue with the promotor directly. For example, if you as a judge are unclear about the sequence of the judging categories, don't understand the scoring sheets or anything else, by all means, speak up!

Promoters go to a great deal of effort to make the contest come off smoothly. Consequently, they deserve the best cooperation from you that is possible. This means that you owe it to them and to the contestants to be on time, every time. Find out when you are supposed to be somewhere and be there by then or even a bit early. Judges, including some famous ones, have been disqualified for late arrival in more than one contest, and this makes everybody uncomfortable. If you must be late, call ahead to warn people who may have to deal with the problems created by your lateness; not to do so is rude.

Usually, contestants and judges are given a badge that

identifies them when they arrive and they are expected to wear it in public until the contest is concluded. This custom has several purposes. It reduces the possibility that judges and contestants might accidentally "play" together before the contest and thereby jeopardize the integrity of the judging result. The badges also make it easier for judges to evaluate contestants in a social setting, and for the contestants to make personal contact with judges. It also tends to prevent people who may be friends of contestants from lobbying a judge in favor of a competitor.

National level judges face another problem that is related to this issue. Just because a contestant you've got your eye on to play with loses in the current contest does not prevent him/her from entering another one in the next town or state where you might be judging again next month or in eight months. If you as a judge have tricked with this contestant, there is always the possibility that somebody might want to make a stink about it. Judges get horny, too! What is the solution?

One way around this is for the judge to drop a question into conversation before going off together for the night: "Why aren't you in this contest? You should enter". If the person has contest aspirations, s/he will often come out with this information in response to your question.

Generally, the more time that passes between the sexual get-together and the contest you have to judge, the safer you are likely to be from charges of favoritism. This situation probably does not come up often, but frequency is not the issue. The integrity of the contest process is what matters. Discretion is called for if you want to be respected as a judge.

Several experienced judges have pointed out that having tricked with a contestant is almost more likely to work against the contestant than in their favor, so judges will sometimes have to remember to not let prior contact negatively prejudice their views of a particular contestant.

It is courteous to drop the promoters and the winners a note when you return home from the contest. In addition to your thanks, you might also want to make any constructive suggestions that occur to you, but do so gently.

As a judge, you have much of the responsibility to the contestants to ensure a fair result. If you think something is about to happen that could compromise the integrity of the contest, you may at any time notify the head judge or any of the senior production staff about your concern or objection.

If, for example, you want some assurances that the scores will be unchanged between prejudging and the public show, you are well within your rights to request that the scores be sealed. Usually, you can solicit support for your idea from the other judges and get it without much of a problem.

Lastly, the title system requires really good judging for it to work well. This means that the contestants deserve your best observation skills and your most careful attention when they are in the midst of competition. Remember, as a judge, you choose on behalf of the community, not just yourself.

HOLDING A TITLE

Following are some thoughts on holding a title. Hopefully, they will give contestants hoping to win a title some things to think about and will help new winners get a grip on some of the issues that confront titleholders all the time.

This section has been written with the international titles in mind, so what follows will not always be relevant on the regional, state or local level. Nevertheless, with some careful reading between the lines, these ideas can be adapted if they suit you and fit with your agenda for your title year.

A Perspective

The privilege is given to only a few to influence and to serve. Titleholding is a very special kind of volunteer service position. From a certain point of view, titleholders are a short-term, quasi-feudal nobility or aristocracy that the leather community has created to serve a number of different functions. Titleholders, as a sort of nobility, rule over no one and have no authority. Here in the democratic world, people have come to be suspicious of all nobility because it has been long associated with oppression, class, special privilege and the like.

When judges confer a title, they encourage the members of our community to extend respect, attention and courtesy to a titled person. Furthermore, the community is also encouraged to accept the titled person as a role model. All this can be lost—forfeited if the titled person fails to continually earn that respect, attention and courtesy. His/her status as a role model depends on behavior.

Over the years, titled persons have always lost their credibility and community respect whenever they were lazy, haughty, condescending, confusing, flip-floppy, hostile, arrogant, petty, mean-spirited, drug/alcohol abusive, over-exposed, uncooperative, demanding, weak, unreliable, or otherwise false or inappropriate. Like most people in public life, titled people are usually held up to standards that are more demanding than the general public measures itself by. This is not necessarily fair, but it is fact.

Even under these pressures, the rewards can be great. The satisfaction that comes from knowing you've done a good job is second to none if you can keep that perspective.

Some Thoughts On Being A "Leather Star"

Twinkle twinkle, little star. How I wonder...

You may or may not have been a star before you won your new title, but you are one now whether you want to be or not. Many leather folks will treat you like a star (whatever that means to them) and, likewise, they will be expecting you to behave like a star.

We all know that the public feels differently about different stars. This happens because there are many ways to be a star, and the public knows this. They watch to see if you behave pompously, or like a kindly monarch, like a confident but humble public servant, or like a porn star who expects everyone to make a pass, or like an average sort of person. Hopefully, you were wise enough to make some decisions before entering the contest about how you wanted to come across in public and can remind yourself about these decisions before you make your appearances.

In general, it is likely that you will get farther with your public and be able to accomplish your objectives more effectively if people find you warm, accessible, ready with a smile, and willing to exchange pleasantries with everyone, if only for a moment. Your style, of course, will be up to you.

There is a time and a place to act like a hot leather icon (usually this is on stage when performing a fantasy or some such) and a time to be "just folks"—these choices are yours. Rest assured that the next year of your life will become public property in some ways, and that even the most private moments have the potential to become very public, depending on how people in the community talk about you and the people you are involved with.

Also be aware that there are lots of leather and non-leather people who don't think much of titleholders for a wide variety of reasons. Some small percentage of these people like to engage titleholders in conversation just to probe for weaknesses or to try to make fools out of them in some way, apparently so that they can continue to justify their condescending attitude toward titleholders as individuals or as titleholders as a class. Watch out for these people and pay attention to your feelings about people's motives when you are dealing with them and you should be able to avoid problems.

The person or organization who sponsored you when you were a contestant does not own you now that you have won. Be careful not to get caught up in the political problems that your former sponsor had or you will risk losing your credibility in the community. Once you win, your important relationship is with the community that you serve. The relationship with your sponsor comes second, especially when they are in conflict.

Photos And Stationery

One thing you should definitely consider doing very early is to order personalized stationery. If your prizes include stationery. I suggest that you don't delay. Order it as soon as you get home. You may find that you already have lots of notes (especially thank-yous) to write from the winning weekend, if that is your style. Note paper and note-sized envelopes, and business cards with your address and phone number, are a good idea and will save you lots of writing time.

It is a good idea that all your leather correspondence be on your official stationery. People will write to you. Some collect notes from all the previous winners and they generally expect you to write to them on something that connects you with your title.

If you plan to make yourself available for fundraisers and other events, it would also be a good idea to write up a press release about yourself and send it off with photos to all the national and regional publications where you might be making appearances in the future. Also, it is from your press release that sponsors get information to publish in their local press to hype their events. You will save yourself and others time, and increase the success of promoters' events, by doing this. It is perfectly reasonable for you to ask your sponsor (if you have one) to underwrite the costs that go with photos and press releases.

Most likely you are in good physical shape right after you win and that is the best time to have photos taken. You may be traveling a lot and that usually means that it is much tougher to stay in good shape. So, think about photos soon.

If you decide to go this route and you think the demand for you will justify the cost, you can usually get by with $200 to $400 for a really good set of photos. You will find that 8x10 glossy photos is what promoters tend to prefer, but 5x7's will usually do just fine.

It is a good idea to have four different images to send to sponsors for their advance publicity and advertising needs if you expect to make appearances in more than, say, four cities. Probably 100 of each image should be enough if you hold a national or international title. If your budget is limited, one or two 5x7 images will do just fine for publicity purposes, but for autographs, the larger ones work much better. Have the photographer or photo reproduction studio be sure to frame your image such that you have room to sign the photos and be sure to have your title and year printed right on the photo across the bottom or down the side.

Have some shots taken with your medal, some with your sash, some with not much on, and some in full leather. Some should be all smiles and others just dripping with sex. Plan ahead. You may want a photo that you can have turned into a greeting card to send out for the holidays. If you do that sort of thing, you will save yourself lots of time if you start your card list now.

Having a stylist with you during the photo shoot who can look after details during the shoot to make sure that the images have as few flaws as possible can be extremely helpful.

Your image is valuable. Try to control which photos of you are given out for publication.

Sometimes you will find that someone takes and publishes a really good photo of you that you like very much. You can track it down and often get permission to use it for your own publicity purposes. Be sure to credit the photographer right on the photo.

In most localities, there is a photographer capable of producing decent photos. If you don't know of one, ask around or contact other titleholders or your sponsor for suggestions.

Giving Your Autograph

It is generally a good idea to carry a pen with you to sign things. When you are asked to give an autograph, it is customary to ask the person, "What's your name, please?" If it can be spelled in more than one way, ask about the spelling. First name is enough unless they specify first and last name.

In general, people like to get more than just your name when you give your autograph. Many titleholders develop several sort of stock things to write when signing something, for example: Yours in fantasy; This is just for John Doe; Thanks for coming tonight, John; or, for a sponsor or bar owner... Thanks for all your help with this contest, you made things lots easier, John; Good to meet you, Richard; Keep on pumpin' iron, fellah; Bottoms up; just to name a few.

When you travel, consider taking along 10 or 20 photographs to sign for people. They really appreciate it. Sponsors of the events you attend will like that, too. Sometimes, photos get auctioned off at fundraising events. Then, it is sometimes nice to write something like, "Thanks for your contribution, it's important..."

Fans want to be able to read what you have written. Write slowly and clearly.

Dealing With Promoters

Promoters will probably contact you and invite you to participate in some event they have organized. Usually the event is a contest, but sometimes it is an anniversary party of a club or organization, a cocktail party, a dance, an auction, etc. Often, these events are fundraisers that have been organized to raise money for a local charity, such as AIDS-related organizations, hospices, counseling centers, local newspapers, crisis hotlines, and others.

The promoter may be a bar owner, representative of a local leather, levi, or motorcycle club, a parade organizer, or production company representative. They may have gotten your phone number from friends, directory assistance, or other sources. Some invitations come in the mail. Sponsors and promoters of local events are a very important community resource and, for that reason, it is a good idea to make sure that things go smoothly during negotiations with these people. Here are some tips —

- Start an event calendar. Don't trust your memory. There will be too many dates to keep track of in your head. Your local stationery store sells inexpensive appointment calendars that work well. Get two of them that are the same except for color, one for home and one to travel with. Update them often so that they both have the same information. If the one you take with you on trips gets lost with your baggage, you still have the copy at home. Otherwise, all that information could be lost and very troublesome to try to reconstruct.

- Decide early in your title year just how much traveling you are willing to do and try hard to stick to your plan. If you try to do too much, you risk burnout and then it all stops being any fun and you might come to resent the title and all that goes with it. On the other hand, if community service is your thing, it is also true that the bigger your title, the bigger your community is.

  Please be sure to make time for yourself. You can't be everywhere. You will very likely have to decline some invitations. Remember, there are other people who can make appearances at events, too. You don't have to do it all. When you must decline, have names and phone numbers to suggest to promoters as alternatives to yourself.

- Resist the temptation to make commitments without your event calendar in front of you. "Thanks for the invitation, but I'm not sure that time isn't already booked. I'll have to get back to you. If you haven't heard from me in a week, please call me. Here is my card." This move buys you time to decide carefully if you want to do the event. It also avoids double-booking—something that really annoys promoters and makes you look disorganized.

- The promoters talk to each other, and word does get around about how you do business. Many of them assume that titleholders are well-networked with each other, and so titleholders sometimes get calls saying, "I tried to reach so-and-so, but he won't return my calls. Would you please contact him and get him to call me because we need a decision from him about such-and-such."

So, please get in the habit of returning phone calls promptly! If you are out of town for an event or getting some rest and relaxation, change your outgoing message on your answering machine so that callers know how long you will be out-of-touch and also when they can expect to hear from you. As a community representative, you are expected to be accessible. No one will mind if you disappear for a few days, but folks get nervous when they think you have dropped out of sight indefinitely.

- Ask about the event: What is the event? What do they want you to do there? (judge, speak, perform, emcee?) Have they done this event before? Have they budgeted money for your plane fare? What plans can they make for your housing? Meals? Ground transportation? Airport pickup? Airport drop-off?

  Experienced promoters are used to these questions, so they will not be surprised when you ask them. After your questions have been answered, you may want to think about them before making a commitment. If you need consultation, don't hesitate to call other titleholders who may know the promoter to talk things over. They may be able to tell you more than the promoter has told you. The well-known titleholders are not hard to track down. The leather magazines can usually help you find them fast.

- If you decide to attend the event, mark your calendar, note the name of the event, name of the promoter, his/her phone numbers and how late you may call in the evening, or how early you may call in the morning. Night or early morning calls are cheaper for you, but be mindful of time zones when making your calls.

If you don't already know, find out what you are expected to do at the event. Get the promoter's address!

- You might even want to send the promoter a note or letter confirming your commitment and detailing your understanding of the arrangements. This can be especially important with respect to finances. This procedure will leave less room for misunderstandings later. Although this sounds very formal, it doesn't have to be.

  In general, it's a good idea to make the travel decisions yourself and then inform the promoter about your ideas before any reservations are made. "I would like to come in on flight 69 on Uranus airlines, which arrives at 4:30 on Friday and leave on flight 122 Sunday afternoon. Will that work for the people picking me up?" When making your travel decisions, be mindful of the fact that sometimes, by taking a slightly earlier or later flight, you can save your host considerable money on air fare.

- It can be a very good idea to send the promoter your photo set and press release when you book the date and suggest that s/he send word of the event to the local gay press with your photo. This will often give the promoter some publicity ideas that may have been missed earlier.

  Sponsors then get the idea that you want to help them make their event a success. When they realize this, they take better care of you and see to it that you are comfortable and have a good time. Everybody is happier that way, and it can feel more like a team effort.

- In your confirmation note, it can be useful to ask for a schedule of events for the weekend, with notations about when and where you are expected to appear, and what you are expected to do there. This helps you plan your time and your wardrobe more smoothly, and avoids the risk that you don't show up when you are expected.

- Consider sending a thank-you note to the promoter and/or housing hosts when you get home after the event. Doing this is not only good manners, it encourages that community to use titleholders in the future and supports the view that we can help and are good role models.

Wearing Medal And Sash

When promoters have paid your way somewhere, they expect you to be visible at their event, and that means flying the flag—wearing your medal, that is. If you weren't awarded a medal, ask your original sponsor to have one made for you so that you have options about what to wear and when. If your sponsor refuses, consider having one made and engraved for yourself (think twice before you reveal this to people if you decide to do so; sponsors don't like to be made to look foolish). Trophy shops will be happy to supply one for small fees.

Also, most titleholders find that when at an event, people like to be able to see a medal. They expect you to wear it, and will often be disappointed not to get a look at it. Some will want to touch it or be photographed with you wearing it. Occasionally, you will find that the medal seems to exert an almost magical effect on some people, almost as if it were a talisman or something.

In general, your title sash is probably best worn when you must be seen from a great distance, like riding in a parade on a float or in an open car. Spend some time in front of a mirror with your sash on to see where it feels best for you. You may have to counter weight it so that it stays put.

Many titleholders feel awkward when wearing sashes, and there is talk among promoters of eliminating them. Perhaps a customized vest or something that can be worn more casually and which does not distance people might be more effective and more tasteful than a sash. Most titleholders prefer to wear their medals rather than their sashes whenever possible. The two times the sash is absolutely required is immediately following the contest for the rest of the evening when in public, and next year when you turn the title over to your successor.

If you are going to a big event (national or international), it is a good idea to pack the sash in case someone wants you to wear it for some special reason. For example, sometimes sponsors will want their winner to be photographed with you in the sash.

The medal will work best for the vast majority of events at which you will be asked to appear. Most titleholders that I have spoken with about this have found that these habits worked best.

At an event where you have to perform any official function (judging, speaking, emceeing a show, running an auction), the medal can be worn hanging around your neck, just above nipple level, or pinned to a vest on one side or the other.

Many contest promoters also present a "title belt" to the winner. Generally, it is best only to wear one symbol at a time, otherwise you can find yourself looking like a billboard trying to draw attention to yourself. There is no one right way to balance wearing these symbols, but "tasteful" should be the watchword.

Tips For Traveling

Traveling is a different experience for everyone. There are ways to make it easier for yourself, and ways to make it hell. If you are planning to travel at every available opportunity, you can look forward to spending lots of time in airports and on planes.

Here are some of the ways you might want to consider that can make it easier for you—

- Join a frequent flyer program right away and remember to give the agent your number whenever making reservations. When you check in at the departure counter on the outbound leg of your trip, double-check to make sure that your frequent flyer number is in the computer. It can be difficult to get milage credit after the trip.

  Consider picking an airline that can be used for almost all your travel so you can accumulate more miles and earn a free trip for yourself as a reward someday, or to attend an important event when no one can pay your way.

- When making reservations, it is a good idea to make reservations as soon as the dates are confirmed with the promoter. Pay for them with your credit card or have the promoters pay on their end. This allows you to reserve good seats for yourself which can make the travel more pleasant. Also, most airlines now offer special meals on most flights. Ask about this when you make reservations. This food, which must be specially ordered, is often much better than the usual fare. If you belong to a frequent flyer program, many airlines offer first class upgrade privilege on a space available basis for a small charge. Check this out before you select your preferred airline.

- There may be times your sponsor wants you to rent a car, so know in advance which car rental companies give you extra miles on your frequent flyer plan. Many airlines offer their own Visa or Mastercard credit card so that when you use it, you add miles to your milage plan. If you go this route, you can charge your air tickets on your card, and ask your hosts to write you a check before leaving their city. You can then apply their check to your card payment. One airline gives miles for using a particular long distance phone service, too, so you might want to shop around for your best deal. During my title year, I accumulated some 95,000 miles.

- It is generally better to have your air tickets sent to you in the mail so that you can check your bags curbside at the airport. Most airlines with curbside baggage check won't check your bags unless you already have a ticket.

- It is strongly suggested that you travel in levis and boots, and either wear or carry your leather jacket and your medal. If your luggage goes to the wrong city, you are still dressed to do the event in a pinch. (The air security people will love your medal!)

- It is also good to carry some sort of folio in which to keep your air ticket and some stationery, including business cards. In this, you might also carry the traveling event calendar because folks always ask where you've been and where you're going next.

Specific information about the particular event you're going to should also be with you in your folio: promoter's name, address and phone number, name of the person picking you up at the airport and their phone number; the name, address and phone number of the place where you are supposed to be first, and the time you are expected there.

Having all this with you can make it possible to function independently even if your luggage gets lost or the pick-up person doesn't show up. Please don't get on a plane without enough money to catch a cab in a pinch.

- Speaking of luggage, I always check all bags to avoid the hassle with carried-on luggage. Only once did I wrestle a set of bags on and off a plane. I was tired from the effort and was not in great form for the first night of the event.

- I use a large, very strong duffel bag for leather, boots, and toys, and a smaller duffel for t-shirts and other washables. There were many times during my title tenure that I did not even unpack the leather bag from weekend to weekend. I just washed the things in the little duffel and repacked it for the next weekend. This saved lots of time and hassle.

- If you performed a fantasy for part of your winning competition, you may be asked to perform it "on-the-road." This may mean extra luggage. Most airlines have a four-bag limit including your two allowable carry-on pieces. If you are going to take a fantasy on the road, you might re-design it to accommodate the needs of travel, or arrange for your needed equipment to be there in the hosting city.

- I always check my bags at curbside because they are heavy with leather, and the skycaps will check practically anything for a tip. A dollar per bag is plenty unless it is extra heavy.

Never try to take kinky equipment onto the plane with you in any carry-on luggage. The security personnel will confiscate handcuffs, whips, pieces of heavy chain, nightsticks, badges, piercing equipment, and the like. This process can make a fuss which can cause you to miss your plane. If you have non-refundable tickets (the cheapest kind), you might not be able to fly if you miss your plane. Kinky gear will travel just fine if you check it.

Some airports are now installing special metal detectors to scan even your checked bags. If you travel with lots of metal gear, they may pull it and make you open it for a closer look. You could have some explaining to do and this might even make you arrive late in the city you are visiting—a complex inconvenience for those picking you up.

The exception to this rule! If you leave the country, kinky gear, porno and uniforms will likely be confiscated at the border and you may be denied entry to the host country. Stuff that is confiscated is usually not returned! Embarrassing. Very expensive and very inconvenient. You can pack rope if you have a good story about why you are bringing it into the country. If you are clever with rope, you can make most anything else you might need for a scene.

If you buy porno of any kind in other countries, be prepared for it to be confiscated at the border when you return to the U.S. Some customs people can be very unpleasant about these things. Border guards can pat you down, tear your car apart and otherwise make your life miserable. Many experienced leather folks choose to dress plainly when crossing borders to avoid the delays that can result when border guards decide to target you with this sort of unwanted attention.

Small Things That Can Make A Big Difference

- A small electric alarm clock (mine prevented me from being late several times).

- A set of those little ear phones that go in your ear (about $25.00). Most wide-body planes have a place to plug them in to your armrest for great sounds at high altitude—maybe a cassette recorder and a favorite tape, too.

- Favorite cold medicines or decongestant sprays.
- Wax or foam ear plugs for the plane or for trying to sleep in a strange house or hotel.
- Eye drops.
- A small penlight (great for judging contests in the dark).
- Fifteen or twenty 8x10 glossy photos and a felt tip pen, just in case.
- Titleholder business cards.
- The name, address and phone number of the promoter tucked away in your wallet.
- If you are used to sleeping in a dark room, take along a sleep mask, available at finer drug stores, unless you want to risk doing an important event on no sleep.

Happy Trails!

About Contests

It will come as no surprise that you will be asked to participate in lots of leather contests, usually as a judge, and sometimes as head judge. At other times, you may be asked to emcee the show, or participate in some other way.

Unfortunately, as often as not, the organizers of contests leave lots of little details (sometimes big ones, too) until the last minute because they have bigger problems on their minds. When this happens, you may sometimes get the feeling that the event is on the verge of spinning out of control, and you may then wish to lend a helping hand.

Often, but not always, local organizers are open to suggestions about how the contest might be run, judged, and scored a bit more smoothly or fairly than promoters had originally planned. As a titleholder, you are sometimes in a position to exert influence on how these things are done if you should choose to do so. The time to consider doing so is when you sense that the promoters are inexperienced about how these things are done and that they would be open to, and perhaps even thankful for, some guidance.

Nothing requires you to take an activist role in these situations, but it won't hurt you to think through the following issues to help you get some clarity about this.

Issues

- To what extent are you willing to become part of the production team?

- Are you willing to make suggestions when you feel that a change might make things come off smoother?

- How good are you at handling potentially delicate egos under the pressure that can go with contest production?

- Do you feel that the success of the event is a reflection on you since you are there as a participant? Do you have an investment in seeing it not fall on its face?

- Do you care whether or not folks come away from the show feeling that the outcome is fixed or rigged in some way? Are you willing to take steps to remove the possibility of this charge being raised?

- Is your willingness to help with the contest determined by whether or not you like the organizers?

- Do you feel any commitment to the contestants? If so, what is the nature of that commitment?

- Have you reached any personal conclusion as to the value of contests to the leather community?

The answers to these questions can help you determine the extent of the role that you might play in contest production as a problem solver or problem identifier.

Always, the big challenge in these situations is how to illuminate for the organizers of the event a potential problem that you may have spotted or that someone else may have privately brought to your attention, perhaps a contestant. Event organizers often have proud and delicate egos that must be respected and supported for the good of the event itself and the community it serves. Such situations will test your best diplomatic abilities.

To be of any value in such situations, you must first have a working knowledge of what makes a well-run contest happen. If you have read all of the foregoing sections, you should have at least a general grasp of the mechanics of these kinds of events. Below is a brief summary of the parts of the leather contest. Consult the previous Production and Judging sections for much more detailed information.

In a sense, there are two different "divisions," so to speak, on the contest circuit. The Mr. Drummer contests (regional and international) constitute one series of contests that are supposed to be run in a more or less standard format that is dictated by the management of Drummer magazine, currently based in San Francisco.

Of the following elements, the Mr. Drummer contests traditionally have the interview, jockstrap/skinshow, fantasy performance, and speech segments. Other sorts of leather contests may have any combination of the parts listed below, but not usually all of them.

- The Interview (if used for eliminations, it is called Prejudging. This usually happens earlier the same day or may happen the day before the main part of the contest. Contestants are usually permitted to wear whatever they wish, although organizers will occasionally specify what is expected.)

- Casual Wear or Street Wear Presentation

- Jockstrap/Skinshow Presentation, also sometimes known as the "Swim Wear" or "Fantasy Wear" segment.

- A Fantasy Performance presentation
- Speech Presentation (often done in "Formal Leather Wear" or "Full Leather Image")
- A Question (read from a card drawn on stage)

A Word About Leadership

Not long ago, it was reported that a new regional titleholder asked for microphone time at a bar event that was scheduled to take place in his town. He apparently felt the obligation to ask for microphone time because he had just become a "community leader." The event organizer casually asked the titleholder what he might say, and the title holder replied with something like, "I want to make an announcement about how anxious I am to honor my leadership responsibilities; if people will just tell me where they want to go, I will lead them."

If leather folks knew where they wanted to go, there would be no need for leadership. This fellow was really saying that he wanted to follow the pack rather than guide it. There is a difference between being a leader and being a figurehead.

While it is valuable to listen to what people want, it is the leader's responsibility to determine the correct path to take, and then to justify and defend that vision. S/he must then inspire others to share his or her journey down that path by taking some definite action.

To determine the correct path, the leader must first have a clear view of the reality of our community circumstances and then couple that view with his or her values with respect to what is nurturing, generative, healthy, liberating, affirming, protective, and otherwise supportive of us in our chosen lifestyle or sexstyle.

The reason that leaders differ in their views (visions) has to do with differences in the clearness with which they see the world as it really is, and also their differences in values about what is good for the leather tribes. For example, some leather leaders feel that it is the task of leadership to inspire leather folks to have a good time and "party hearty" as a way of dealing with the sadness and loss that have racked our community. Others see value in seeking our rightful place among the other erotic minorities, and so forth.

To be truly a leader will require you to first try to see the world and our situation in it with as much clarity as you can. Second, determine your values as to what is really important and will add to who we are as individuals and as a community. Third, clarify for yourself how these two views go together. Fourth, have the courage of your convictions, and speak the truth about them. Fifth, be open to new information about the world and its realities so that you can change your vision of the right path as you learn more. Finally, to allow for the possibility that other leaders can hold a different view without necessarily being in opposition to yours.

If you didn't give serious thought to the nature of leadership before you entered the contest you won, now is an excellent time to do that. The judges probably chose you the winner because of your potential for leadership as well as for your suitability as a figurehead. As a figurehead, you may discover that you either do or do not wish to become (or remain) a leader. This is a choice, and it is yours now.

A Meditation About Glory

At the end of the feature film, Patton, I seemed to recall a kind of voice-over epilogue spoken by George C. Scott which recounted the fact that Roman conquerors received a triumphal parade upon their return to Rome. The returning hero rode in a chariot through the streets of the city, prisoners walking in chains before him. But standing just behind the hero in the chariot was a slave who held a golden laurel wreath above the conquerors head, all the while whispering into his ear the warning: all glory is fleeting.

Try to remember that your year will end one day, and that you will have to learn about a graceful retirement, and re-define some of your connections to those who knew you before you won, and will know you after you have stepped down. The glory will fade, and satisfaction with your accomplishments will come to replace it if you have done your job well.

CONCLUSION

The leather title network has been inaccessible to most folks because it has been something that very few people really knew much about. If the title system is going to be fully usable by our community, then more people need to understand how it works and how it does not work and what its limitations are. I hope this little book sheds light on the system's inner workings and serves to de-mystify it.

I wish this book had been written years ago, and I recognize the fact that in some ways, it is arrogant of me to have done so now. The guide is not complete and, perhaps, never will be, but it is a start. Hopefully, as more and more people read it, comments will flow in and future editions will be improved. Your input can be directed to Guy Baldwin, c/o Daedalus Publishing Company, 2140 Hyperion Avenue, Los Angeles, CA 90027 USA,

I remain…

Your servant in leather,
Guy Baldwin

APPENDIX

Appendix A	Sample Memo to Contestants from Contest Promoter
Appendix B	Sample Memo to Judges from Contest Promoter
Appendix C	Sample Judging Form
Appendix D	Sample Score Elimination Form (Olympic Scoring)
Appendix E	Sample Judging Procedures and Rules
Appendix F	Sample Staging Information for Contestants
Appendix G	Sample Judging Outline
Appendix H	Sample Contestant Schedule
Appendix I	Sample Press Release
Appendix J	Sample Fantasy Script
Appendix K	Sample Prop List for Fantasy
Appendix L	Sample Stage Layout for Fantasy

APPENDIX A

[Promoter's Letterhead]

TO: Contestants
FROM: Mr./Ms. Promoter
CC: Judges, Contest Staff, Sponsors

Enclosed you will find a copy of a memo of instructions to the judges for this contest. If you read it carefully, you will know what is expected of you as a contestant in this contest and the specific criteria you will be judged on.

The contestant application and model release that you have signed outlines some of the expectations and requirements you will have as Mr./Ms. [contest name] should you win. This memo will serve to reiterate those expectations and requirements and also fill you in on more specifics about this contest.

During the year in which the winner holds their title, we hope they will be an able spokesperson for the leather/SM/fetish community. Although you are not required to do so, we hope, should you win, you will make yourself available as much as possible to events including contests, shows, and other places where leather men and women gather. Throughout your title year we hope you will promote diversity of lifestyle and erotic expression and encourage cooperation among the various elements of our community. We also hope you will keep yourself informed on the various issues that are of importance to the leather/SM/fetish community.

However, we understand that to appear at many of these events takes money and that your financial resources may be limited. We do not expect you to go broke in the process of fulfilling your obligations as Mr./Ms. [contest name]. Perhaps the prize money given in this contest to the first place winner will assist in various travel and appearance expenses.

In addition to personal appearances, you may be offered many opportunities to earn money through photo shoots, videos, and other kinds of performance and endorsements. We hope the winner will participate in as many of these opportunities as possible and will use those receipts towards other personal appearance expenses.

We hold our titleholders in the highest regard and feel others should also. Our winner should expect to have their airfare and accommodations paid for by the host business or organization. But many of the requests will come from worthwhile non-profit organizations. When possible, we hope you can arrange to offer your services without financially burdening their cause. Once again, though, this title should not be an undue financial burden on you either. Use your best judgment in these matters. When confronted with many conflicting choices, your decision will have to be based on which event you believe will serve the community best as well as your availability and the financial arrangements.

If for some reason the winner is unable to carry out their title responsibilities due to job, health, geographics, or other personal reasons, we expect that person to pass their title on to the first runner up.

We would appreciate it if the winner would also keep a record of their activities as titleholder. This will be used to further promote you as titleholder and serve as a way for us to know which businesses and organizations hold our title in high enough regard to request the winner's presence.

Thanks for your participation in this contest. We will do everything in our power to make the experience an enjoyable one.

APPENDIX B

[Promoter's Letterhead]

TO: Judges
FROM: Mr./Ms. Promoter
CC: Contestants, Contest Staff, Sponsors

Judges, you have an important task to undertake. In a few weeks, contestants will be vying for our title and it is your job to pick the winners. This memo outlines what type of person we hope will represent this title and the judging criteria to be used.

Our winner should be a person who can and will be an active and positive representative of the leather/SM community. Along with other leather titleholders, they should be a positive role model for other leather men and women.

Intelligence, personality and an articulate style are all important. A good physical presence and the ability to hold people's attention through words and deeds are desirable traits. Our winner should have energy, initiative, and the time to put their talents to use. And yes, our winner should be erotic and hot, but that should not take precedence over other qualities. They should also have enough experience to command respect as a leader, but even more important, they should be willing and eager to learn from the experience of others.

You will score the contestants five times. Once during individual interview sessions on Saturday morning and four more times during the contest on Saturday evening. The maximum total score is 1000 points. Please score in increments of 5 points only (105, 310, 595, etc.). Once you have scored each of the five appearances you will pass that score sheet on to the person assigned to tally the scores. You can not change the score after it is given to the person tallying.

You are judging the contestants on the basis of personality, physical appearance, and leather image (whatever that means to you). These categories are not scored separately, but they should be kept in mind when doing the scoring.

All judging will take place at the Main Street Theater which is located at 1234 Main Street, Anywhere, Anycity. The phone number there is (123) 456-7890 (use for emergencies only).

Important: Don't forget to give your score sheet to the tally person after every judging session.

Interview: 300 points maximum—On Saturday, beginning at 10 a.m., the panel of judges will meet with each contestant. You may ask whatever questions you wish. The alternate judge may participate in the questioning and should score the event too. This is, perhaps, one of the most important judging sessions. You should score for intelligence, grasp of issues, personality, ability to communicate and general ability to fulfill the responsibilities of the title. Each judge should score privately, but it is permissible for the judges to discuss the contestant amongst themselves (do this only when the contestant has left the room and no other contestants are present).

You may have up to 10 minutes with each contestant. Be aware that they probably will not appear in numerical order as they will be scheduled as they have time free from rehearsals. The head judge will serve as moderator for this panel. Don't forget to turn in your score sheets to the tally person. Score sheets will be sealed in your presence and the head judge will sign their name across the seal.

Opening Comments: 100 points maximum—Each contestant, dressed in casual or cruising attire of their choice, will be introduced to the audience, will walk the runway, and will have an opportunity to make a brief (1 minute maximum) opening remark. In your scoring consider appearance and general stage presence. Pass your score sheet to the tally person.

Fantasy: 300 points maximum—Each contestant, with or without assistance from others, will perform a fantasy presentation. In scoring, consider the originality and creativity of the skit and consider the balance between erotic intensity and the message being communicated to the audience.

The first set of contestants will present their fantasies followed by an intermission and the jock strap presentation. Then, the remaining contestants will present their fantasies. Retain your score sheet until all fantasies have been presented. Please keep them protected and confidential during the intermission. Pass them to the tally person after the last fantasy.

Jock Strap/Brief Attire: 200 points maximum—Each contestant

will walk the runway. Naturally, for this event, physical appearance should be the prime criteria in scoring. Pass your sheets to the tally person when completed.

Final Parade/Question: 100 points maximum—Each contestant will be individually introduced and walk the runway dressed in his "leather image" attire. This should set the tone of the image he wishes to present as winner of the title. Before leaving the stage the contestant will be asked a question selected at random from a prepared list. This is your last look and your last opportunity to score the contestants. Pass your completed score sheets on to the tally person.

Tabulations: The tally person will compute the final score awarded by each of the judges to each of the contestants. A modified Olympic scoring system will be used, meaning that the highest and lowest scores for each contestant will be eliminated and the remaining five scores added together for a maximum possible 5000 points. I and my assistant will review the numbers with the tally person. The contestant receiving the highest number of points will be the winner. Next highest will be first runner up and next highest second runner up. The tally person and I will keep the results confidential until they are announced from the stage.

Judges score sheets will be identified only by a code, not the judge's name. I will have the only key to that code. The tally person will turn the judge's score sheets and the final tally sheet over to me immediately following the contest. These will be available for review by any judge, contestant, or sponsor wishing to do so. Anyone wishing to review the sheets should make the request directly to me.

The Alternate Judge: The Alternate Judge will participate in the interview sessions and will score these. If one of the other judges fails to participate in these sessions, the scores of the alternate judge will be included in the final tabulations. Should one of the judges fail to participate in the scoring at the contest itself the alternate judge will substitute for him and his scores for the interview will be used instead of those of the judge he replaces. Should more than one of the regular judges fail to participate, or should the alternate fail to participate, I will select an additional alternate judge.

APPENDIX C

JUDGING FORM

Judge #1				
Contestant	Interview 0-100 pts.	Casual Wear 0-40 pts.	Brief Attire 0-40 pts.	Full Leather Speech 0-80 pts.
1				
2				
3				
4				
5				
6				
7				
8				
9				
10				
11				
12				
13				
14				
15				
16				
17				
18				

APPENDIX D

ELIMINATION FORM—INTERVIEW SEGMENT

OLYMPIC SCORING

<u>INTERVIEW</u>

0 - 100 points

Contestant	Judge 1	Judge 2	Judge 3	Judge 4	Judge 5	Judge 6	Judge 7	Total

APPENDIX E

JUDGING PROCEDURES AND RULES

The official Olympic Scoring will be used for totalling points. In order to insure the utmost fairness in selecting the winners of this contest, the official Olympic Scoring System, the same method used in the Olympic Games, will be used when totalling each contestant's points. This will help to eliminate any unfairness or favoritism.

Contestants will be judged in three categories for a total of 0 to 100 points. The categories are:

The Leather Image	0 to 40 points
Physical Appearance	0 to 30 points
Attitude and Personality	0 to 30 points

In the first parade of contestants, all contestants will appear in an outfit of their choice. No scoring should be done at this time. During the second parade of contestants, the contestants will appear in swimsuit or similar attire. Scoring for Physical Appearance should be done at this time. During the third parade of contestants, the contestants will appear in their leather outfit and will be given one and a half minutes to introduce themselves. It is at this time that scoring should be done in the Attitude/Personality and Leather Image categories.

Keep in mind that what you are looking for is not necessarily the most attractive face or the hottest body, but rather the person who best typifies the ideal of leather to you; someone whose poise and self-assurance, whose very presence is imbued with that special and unidentifiable quality we recognize as "Leather."

APPENDIX F

STAGING INFORMATION FOR CONTESTANTS

Parade of Contestants (Dress: Total Leather) (Semi-Finalists)
10:45 p.m. (on stage)
Judging: Total leather image and attitude/personality.

A. Line up in numerical order backstage.
B You will be introduced one at a time. Walk to position #1 (center stage), then to position #2 (front center stage), then back to the microphone at position #1. Your statement to the audience may concern any aspect of leather, the community, or your image should you win this contest. You may not exceed 1½ minutes. In order to give everyone equal time, your microphone will be cut off exactly 1½ minutes after you begin speaking.
C. Do not leave position #1 until the emcee's dismiss you. Important!—The judges are scoring you for the final time now—do not leave the stage until the emcee's release you, since that signal reaches the emcee's via the judges.
D. When dismissed, exit stage right.
E. Line up again backstage to walk the stage a final time with the rest of the semi-finalists.

Awards Presentations (Dress: Total Leather) (Semi-Finalists)
12:10 a.m. (on stage)

A. All semi-finalists line up backstage when directed.
B. On cue from the Production Manager, enter the stage in formation and go to your pre-assigned position on stage.
C. Wait.
D. If you are selected, please stand on the appropriate winner's box. The order of awards is: second runner up, first runner up, winner.
E. All semi-finalists remain on the stage for photographs, until you are released by the Production Manager.
F. When dismissed, return to the dressing rooms (the three winners will remain on stage for additional photographs).

APPENDIX G

JUDGING OUTLINE

The contestants will be judged in the following five categories:

1. Prejudging: A meeting will be held between the judges and each contestant. This will be a time for the judges to meet and talk with the contestant.

2. Street Clothes: This will be the first presentation of the contestants to the audience. Each contestant will be given 30 seconds of mike time to express why they wish to win this contest and why they feel they should.

3. Brief Attire: Each contestant will appear in jock strap, swim wear, or other similar attire as part of a staged production number that will double as entertainment for the audience and a chance for judges to score physical appearance.

4. Fantasy: Each contestant enacts a short erotic fantast skit of no more than 5 minutes in length. Prerecorded music and portable props are to be furnished by each contestant. Assistants are allowed. Illegal acts are not allowed and sex acts, if part of the fantasy, should be simulated.

5. Dress Leather: Each contestant is introduced wearing their dress leather. During this presentation, each contestant is to respond to a question drawn from those questions submitted by each contestant.

SCORING

The Olympic Scoring System will be used. Each judge will award 0 to 200 points in each of the above categories. Keep in mind at all times physical appearance, attitude, personality, and leather image. The lowest and highest scores are eliminated. After this elimination the remaining scores are added together. The highest total score is the winner.

APPENDIX H

SCHEDULE OF EVENTS

Friday	8:00 p.m. - 10:30 p.m. Reception for last year's winner. This is a non-judging event.
Saturday	1:00 p.m. - 3:30 p.m. Rehearsal for contestants (Main Street Theater, 1234 Main Street). Please have the music for your fantasy on a cassette tape and all props you will need for the evening at this time.
	3:30 p.m. - 5:00 p.m. Pre-judging interviews (Main Street Theater, 1234 Main Street). Contestants will be interviewed by the judges. When you are not being interviewed you will be scheduled for stage rehearsal time for your fantasy.
	7:15 p.m. All contestants should report backstage (Main Street Theater, 1234 Main Street).
	8:00 p.m. Contest show begins. In your contestant information packet you have a detailed outline of the contest, but a brief synopsis is: Presentation of colors, Dedication, Street Clothes, Brief Attire, Break, Fantasies, Break, Dress Leather, Entertainment, Awards presentation.
Sunday	Winner's breakfast Farewell party (Spike, 3456 Main Street).

APPENDIX I

[Promoter's Letterhead]

For Immediate Release... Contact: Mr./Ms. Promoter
(123) 456-7890

Our city will play host to over 1,000 leathermen, leatherwomen, and their friends during the [contest name] contest to be held on [date].

The winner of this contest will be chosen on the basis of attitude, personality, leather image, community awareness, physical appearance, and speaking ability. The goal is to choose the person with the best overall set of qualities rather than necessarily the one with the most attractive appearance.

This contest is produced by the men and women of United People of Leather, an organization dedicated to the betterment of the leather lifestyle in our city. All profits from the contest will be donated to the Children's Research Hospital and our city's Gay and Lesbian Community Services Center.

The festivities will begin Friday of that weekend with a welcome party for all contestants and other interested folks at the Spike, located at 3456 Main Street. All are welcome to this party, whether attending the contest or not.

On Saturday the contest will be held at 8:00 p.m. at the Main Street Theater, 1234 Main Street. The audience will be treated to a stage full of attractive leatherfolks vying for the title as well as a variety of scheduled entertainment.

The Spike will host a victory party for the winner on Sunday evening at 9:00 p.m. All are invited.

Tickets for the contest are $10.00 in advance and $15.00 at the door. They can be purchased in advance at the Spike, at the Leather Shop, 5678 Main Street, or by mail. If interested, you can call the contest information line for a recorded message of up-to-the-minute contest news and ticket information at (123) 456-7890.

APPENDIX J

FANTASY SCRIPT

BLACKOUT STAGE

CUE: MUSIC UP SLOWLY. FULL STAGE DAYLIGHT. AFTER 5 SECONDS OF MUSIC—

Boy enters from right, crosses first to mirror (full size frame fitted with taut, vertically stretched plastic wrap), looks at self in mirror, fusses with hair, then crosses to bed in bedroom stage left, sets alarm clock on nightstand, sits on bed, removes clothing to white underwear, turn down bed linen. Boy gets into bed, reaches back and turns out lamp.

CUE: INSTANT FLOOD STAGE WITH BLUE LIGHT ONLY

Boy "goes to bed," but doesn't sleep well. Boy tosses and turns as if in a dream/nightmare for a moment or two.

CUE: SINGLE, BIG SMOKE PUFF UP FROM BEHIND BOY'S BED

Bodybuilder wearing similar style of white underwear appears in smoke (standing on a box hidden behind the bed) and executes a posing routine for 30 seconds, then disappears back behind the bed.

CUE: BLUE LIGHT SLOWLY REPLACED WITH FULL DAYLIGHT

CUE: ALARM CLOCK GOES OFF

Boy turns off clock, gets out of bed and grabs two dumbbells and begins to pump his biceps while walking around the stage, stopping in front of mirror. As he steps in front of mirror, bodybuilder steps simultaneously into place behind "mirror" (plastic wrap) and begins to match the movements of the boy.

Boy continues pumping arms with weights, but turns around to face audience (his back is to the mirror).

Bodybuilder puts his weights down, feels the "mirror" from the inside searching for a way "through" the mirror, finds a seam and spreads the mirror open, steps through it and up behind the boy who is still pumping the weights, but facing the audience.

Bodybuilder grabs boy, boy drops weights, bodyworship happens, bodybuilder throws boy over shoulder and carries boy back through mirror.

CUE: INSTANT FADE TO BLACK AS THEY EXIT THROUGH THE MIRROR.

APPENDIX K

PROP LIST FOR FANTASY

1. Single bed with bed linen, one large blanket hangs down touching stage.

2. Nightstand next to bed with lamp and large alarm clock (electric).

3. "Mirror" (large size frame, 7'x3' is ideal) which has been stretched with plastic wrap vertically (an overlap seam down the center) which stands securely on the stage.

4. Two sets of 10-12 lb. dumbbells (one set is bedside, the other hidden behind the "mirror."

5. One box (milk crate okay) behind bed for bodybuilder to stand on during posing routine.

6. Smoke machine.

7. Muscle magazine (prepare with photo of bodybuilder in fantasy, if possible, on the cover).

APPENDIX L

STAGE LAYOUT FOR FANTASY

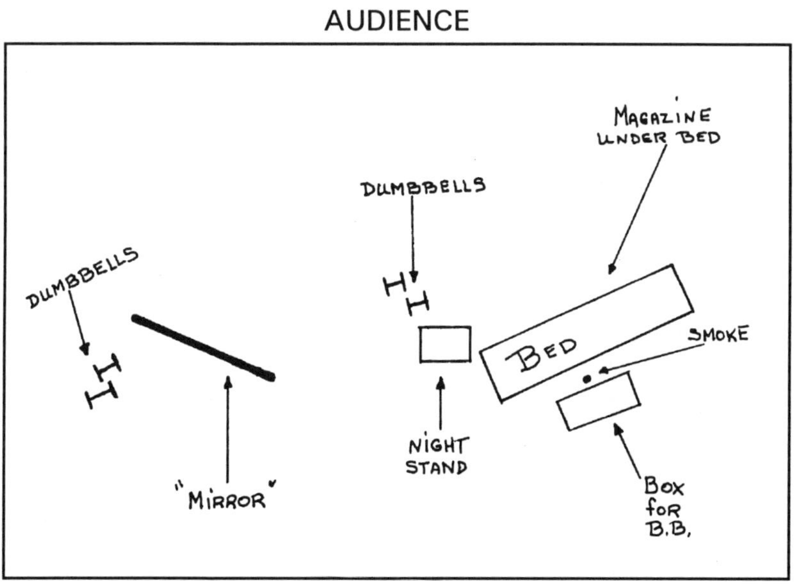

ABOUT THE AUTHOR

A Los Angeles-based psychotherapist and author, Guy Baldwin, has worked professionally with leather folks for the last 20 years. An active player himself in the Scene for 37 years, Guy has traveled the US and Canada extensively to present a wide array of workshops, demonstrations, seminars and lectures, to leather audiences and health-care professionals alike. He has delivered keynote addresses for the Leather Leadership Conference, the Dominion Gathering, the Living in Leather convention of the National Leather Association, the Austin Bash, and the International Masters and slaves weekend.

He is perhaps best known for his essays in *Drummer* magazine, many of which appear in his 1993 book, *Ties That Bind.* His 2002 book, *SlaveCraft* offers a penetrating look into the inner dynamics of erotic servitude. In 1989, Guy served as *International Mr. Leather*, and as *Mister National Leather Association* concurrently.....the only person ever to do so. He was awarded both the *Pantheon* and *Dominion* Lifetime Achievement Awards, and was named a *Centurian* by the Leather Archives and Museum.

Also available from Daedalus Publishing Company

www.daedaluspublishing.com

Painfully Obvious

An Irreverent & Unauthorized Manual for Leather/SM

Robert Davolt's new anthology takes an unorthodox look at leather relationships, community, contests, business, tradition, history and leadership. Inside perspective and practical tips on "What To Wear," "Leather On The Cheap" and "Passing The Bar," are delivered with authoritative research and barbed humor. **$16.95**

Spirit + Flesh

Fakir Musafar's Photo Book

After 50 years photographing Fakir Musafar's own body and the play of others, here is a deluxe retrospective collection of amazing images you'll find nowhere else... 296 oversize pages, three pounds worth! This book is a "must have" for all serious body modifiers, tattoo and piercing studios. **$49.50**

Urban Aboriginals

A Celebration of Leathersexuality – 20th Anniversary Edition

As relevant today as when it was written 20 years ago, author Geoff Mains takes an intimate view of the gay male leather community. Explore the spiritual, sexual, emotional, cultural and physiological aspects that make this "scene" one of the most prominent yet misunderstood subcultures in our society. **$15.95**

Carried Away

An s/M Romance

In david stein's first novel, steamy Leathersex is only the beginning when a cocky, jaded bottom and a once-burned Master come together for some no-strings bondage and s/M. Once the scene is over, a deeper hunger unexpectedly awakens, and they begin playing for much higher stakes. **$19.95**

Ties That Bind

The SM/Leather/Fetish Erotic Style

Issues, Commentaries and Advice

The early writings of well-known psychotherapist and respected member of the leather community Guy Baldwin have been compiled to create this SM classic. Second edition. **$16.95**

SlaveCraft

Roadmaps for Erotic Servitude Principles, Skills and Tools

Guy Baldwin, author of *Ties That Bind*, joins forces with a grateful slave to produce this gripping and personal account on the subject of consensual slavery. **$15.95**

The Master's Manual

A Handbook of Erotic Dominance

In this book, author Jack Rinella examines various aspects of erotic dominance, including s/M, safety, sex, erotic power, techniques and more. The author speaks in a clear, frank, and nonjudgmental way to anyone with an interest in the erotic Dominant/submissive dynamic. **$15.95**

The Compleat Slave

Creating and Living and Erotic Dominant/submissive Lifestyle

In this highly anticipated follow up to The Master's Manual, author Jack Rinella continues his in-depth exploration of Dominant/submissive relationships. **$15.95**

Learning the Ropes

A Basic Guide to Fun S/M Lovemaking

This book, by s/M expert Race Bannon, guides the reader through the basics of safe and fun s/M. Negative myths are dispelled and replaced with the truth about the kind of s/M erotic play that so many adults enjoy. **$12.95**

My Private Life

Real Experiences of a Dominant Woman

Within these pages, the author, Mistress Nan, allows the reader a brief glimpse into the true private life of an erotically dominant woman. Each scene is vividly detailed and reads like the finest erotica, but knowing that these scenes really occurred as written adds to the sexual excitement they elicit. **$14.95**

Consensual Sadomasochism

How to Talk About It and How to Do It Safely

Authors William A. Henkin, Ph. D. and Sybil Holiday, CCHT combine their extensive professional credentials with deep personal experience in this unique examination of erotic consensual sadomasochism. Second edition. **$17.95**

Chainmale: 3SM

A Unique View of Leather Culture

Author Don Bastian brings his experiences to print with this fast paced account of one man's experience with his own sexuality and eventual involvement in a loving and successful three-way kink relationship. **$13.95**

Leathersex

A Guide for the Curious Outsider and the Serious Player

Written by renowned s/M author Joseph Bean, this book gives guidance to one popular style of erotic play which the author calls 'leathersex'- sexuality that may include s/M, bondage, role playing, sensual physical stimulation and fetish, to name just a few. Second edition. **$16.95**

Leathersex Q&A

Questions About Leathersex and the Leather Lifestyle Answered

In this interesting and informative book, author Joseph Bean answers a wide variety of questions about leathersex sexuality. Each response is written with the sensitivity and insight only someone with a vast amount of experience in this style of sexuality could provide. **$16.95**

Beneath The Skins

The New Spirit and Politics of the Kink Community

This book by Ivo Dominguez, Jr. examines the many issues facing the modern leather/SM/ fetish community. This special community is coming of age, and this book helps to pave the way for all who are a part of it. **$12.95**

Leather and Latex Care

How to Keep Your Leather and Latex Looking Great

This concise book by Kelly J. Thibault gives the reader all they need to know to keep their leather and latex items in top shape. While clothing is the focus of this book, tips are also given to those using leather and latex items in their erotic play. This book is a must for anyone investing in leather or latex. **$10.95**

Between The Cracks

The Daedalus Anthology of Kinky Verse

Editor Gavin Dillard has collected the most exotic of the erotic of the poetic pantheon, from the fetishes of Edna St. Vincent Millay to the howling of Ginsberg, lest any further clues be lost *between the cracks*. **$18.95**

Ordering Information

By phone: 323.666.2121
By via email: order@DaedalusPublishing.com
By mail:

Daedalus Publishing Company
2140 Hyperion Ave
Los Angeles, CA 90027

Payment: All major credit cards are accepted. Via *email or regular mail*, indicate type of card, card number, expiration date, name of cardholder as shown on card, and billing address of the cardholder. Also include the mailing address where you wish your order to be sent. Orders via regular mail may include payment by money order or check, but may be held until the check clears. Make checks or money orders payable to "Daedalus Publishing Company." *Do not send cash.*

Tax and shipping California residents, add 8.25% sales tax to the total price of the books you are ordering. *All* orders should include a $4.25 shipping charge for the first book, plus $1.00 for each additional book added to the total of the order.

Since many of our publications deal with sexuality issues, please include a signed statement that you are at least 21 years of age with any order. Also include such a statement with any email order.